Recent Advances in Hypertension, Hypercholesterolemia and Type 2 Diabetes

Recent Advances in Hypertension, Hypercholesterolemia and Type 2 Diabetes

Guest Editor

Tomislav Bulum

MDPI

Basel • Beijing • Wuhan • Barcelona • Belgrade • Novi Sad • Cluj • Manchester

Guest Editor
Tomislav Bulum
Vuk Vrhovac Univerity Clinic
Merkur University Hospital
Zagreb
Croatia

Editorial Office
MDPI AG
Grosspeteranlage 5
4052 Basel, Switzerland

This is a reprint of the Special Issue, published open access by the journal *Biomedicines* (ISSN 2227-9059), freely accessible at: https://www.mdpi.com/journal/biomedicines/special_issues/10J6FV3S54.

For citation purposes, cite each article independently as indicated on the article page online and as indicated below:

Lastname, A.A.; Lastname, B.B. Article Title. *Journal Name* **Year**, *Volume Number*, Page Range.

ISBN 978-3-7258-6766-0 (Hbk)
ISBN 978-3-7258-6767-7 (PDF)
https://doi.org/10.3390/books978-3-7258-6767-7

Contents

About the Editor

Tomislav Bulum

Tomislav Bulum is employed at the Vuk Vrhovac University Clinic for Diabetes, Endocrinology, and Metabolic Diseases, University Hospital Merkur, Croatia's Referral Center for Diabetes, where he currently serves as a Specialist in Internal Medicine and a Subspecialist in Endocrinology and Diabetology. He received his PhD in 2010 from the Faculty of Science, University of Zagreb. Since 2016, he has been employed at the Medical School, University of Zagreb, where he currently holds the position of Associate Professor and Scientific Adviser. He lectures undergraduate courses as well as postgraduate specialist and PhD studies in biomedicine and health sciences at the Medical School, University of Zagreb. He has participated in multiple scientific and clinical projects in the field of type 1 and type 2 diabetes, with a particular focus on chronic diabetic complications.

He has authored over 100 scientific papers published in Web of Science, Scopus, and Index Medicus-indexed journals, as well as over 100 scientific and professional abstracts, with his work cited over 1,000 times. He has served as a Guest Editor for over 10 Special Issues in first-quartile (Q1) journals, including *Biomedicines*, *Journal of Clinical Medicine*, *International Journal of Molecular Sciences*, *Diagnostics*, *Frontiers in Endocrinology*, and *Biology*. In 2023, he received the annual award from the Croatian Medical Chamber for scientific advancement in medicine and professional excellence. He is a member of the Croatian Academy of Medical Sciences.

biomedicines

MDPI

Article

Systolic and Diastolic Blood Pressure Are Independent Risk Factors for Diabetic Retinopathy in Patients with Type 2 Diabetes

Tomislav Bulum [1,2,*], Martina Tomić [3], Romano Vrabec [3], Neva Brkljačić [4] and Spomenka Ljubić [1,2]

1 Department of Diabetes, Vuk Vrhovac University Clinic for Diabetes, Endocrinology and Metabolic Diseases, Merkur University Hospital, 10000 Zagreb, Croatia
2 Medical School, University of Zagreb,10000 Zagreb, Croatia
3 Department of Ophthalmology, Vuk Vrhovac University Clinic for Diabetes, Endocrinology and Metabolic Diseases, Merkur University Hospital, 10000 Zagreb, Croatia
4 Department of Cardiology, Vuk Vrhovac University Clinic for Diabetes, Endocrinology and Metabolic Diseases, Merkur University Hospital, 10000 Zagreb, Croatia
* Correspondence: tomobulum@gmail.com

Abstract: Background and aims: Diabetic retinopathy (DR) is a microvascular complication of diabetes and represents the leading cause of blindness in working-age adults. The aim of this study was to investigate the risk factors for DR in patients with type 2 diabetes (T2DM) with and without diabetic nephropathy (DN). Methods: A total of 160 patients with T2DM were included in the study. Photodocumented retinopathy status was determined according to the EURODIAB protocol. Renal function was determined using creatinine-based estimated glomerular filtration rate (eGFR) and albumin-to-creatinine ratio (ACR). Binary univariate and multiple logistic regression analyses were performed to determine the main predictors of DR. Results: The prevalence of DR in this studied sample was 46.3%. No significant correlation was observed between DR and age, body mass index, serum lipids, and renal function. Binary logistic regression analysis (no DR/DR) showed that longer diabetes duration ($p = 0.008$), poor glycemic control (HbA1c) ($p = 0.008$), higher systolic blood pressure ($p = 0.001$), and diastolic blood pressure ($p = 0.003$) were the main predictors of DR in patients with T2DM. However, the influence of systolic blood pressure (AOR = 1.06, $p = 0.004$) and diastolic blood pressure (AOR = 1.12, $p = 0.007$) on DR development remained significant even after adjustment for diabetes duration and HbA1c. Conclusions: Our results suggest that systolic and diastolic blood pressure are independent risk factors for DR in patients with T2DM.

Keywords: type 2 diabetes; diabetic retinopathy; risk factors; systolic blood pressure; diastolic blood pressure

1. Introduction

The dramatic increase in the prevalence of diabetes mellitus and its complications positions this metabolic disorder as the most common non-communicable disease worldwide. It is estimated that about 700 million people worldwide by 2045 will have diabetes [1]. Despite new therapeutic options, there has also been an increase in chronic complications of diabetes [2]. Diabetic retinopathy (DR) is one of the major chronic complications of diabetes and still represents the leading vision-threatening disease in working-age adults [3]. In prospective studies, hyperglycemia and hypertension have been documented as the most important modifiable risk factors for developing DR, along with the duration of diabetes as the most important non-modifiable risk factor [4–7]. Most patients (about 90%) have type 2 diabetes (T2DM), in which overweight and abdominal obesity plays a crucial role in developing insulin resistance and diabetes. Abdominal obesity and insulin resistance are underlying conditions in developing metabolic syndrome-associated disorders like hypertension and dyslipidemia, which are connected with microvascular complications of diabetes, including DR [8].

The two most common microvascular complications in patients with T2DM are DR and diabetic nephropathy (DN). Since these two microvascular complications share a similar pathogenesis, they are supposed to develop in parallel in patients with diabetes, and the presence and severity of DR are accompanied by the presence and severity of DN [9,10]. However, DR and DN are more closely related and simultaneously progress in patients with type 1 diabetes than in patients with T2DM [11]. The reason could be that at the time of diagnosis of type 1 diabetes, most patients had neither DR nor DN, and over time and with complications development, there are more substantial effects of risk factors associated with DN, like hypertension, on DR development [12]. In T2DM, there is a well-recognized association between DR and DN—DN without DR is rare, but DR without DN is common. DR is associated with an increased risk of DN in patients with T2DM, and the predictive value of DR on subsequent DN risk for T2DM patients is relatively lower [13].

In addition to high blood glucose, blood pressure is also a significant risk factor for the development of DR because high blood pressure is transferred into retinal circulation, leading to injury of retinal endothelial cells [14]. The results from the large and prospective United Kingdom Prospective Diabetes Study (UKPDS) suggest that the risk of DR is increased in patients with T2DM and higher systolic blood pressure (SBP) compared to those with normal blood pressure [15]. Similar outcomes were found in a meta-analysis that included over 100,000 participants, where a decrease in SBP by 10 mmHg reduced the risk of DR by 13% [16]. Generally, there is a high prevalence of hypertension in patients with T2DM because at the time of diagnosis, around 40% of them have high blood pressure, and with increased age and the longer duration of diabetes, the percentage increases—up to 60% in those aged 75. Even in those with SBP < 140 mmHg and diastolic blood pressure (DBP) < 90 mmHg, there is a significant association between SBP and DR after adjusting for known risk factors like hemoglobin A_1c, diabetes duration, and gender [17]. We previously described in T2DM the connection between hypertension and cataract development and the association between systolic blood pressure and the development and progression of DR in patients with type 1 diabetes with normal renal function (normoalbuminuria and estimated glomerular filtration rate over 60 mL/min/1.73 m^2) [18,19].

The aim of this study was to explore the prevalence of DR and DN and risk factors for DR in patients with T2DM with and without DN.

2. Methods

2.1. Study Design and Ethics Statement

Our study was cross-sectional and performed between 15 December 2020 and 15 March 2021 at the Department of Diabetes, Department of Ophthalmology, and Department of Cardiology. The study was conducted following the Declaration of Helsinki and approved by the Hospital's Ethics Committee (protocol number 05/01-849, approval date: 16 September 2020). Before any procedures and inclusion in the study, patients received written and oral information about the study and finally signed informed consent. All patients in the study agreed that their data and image documents could be used for publication in scientific and professional journals.

2.2. Patients

The study included a total of 160 patients with T2DM attending all three Departments on the same day. Patients with illnesses affecting eye and renal function or blood pressure, inflammatory diseases, or acute infectious diseases, and patients who were pregnant or had other forms of eye diseases were not included in the study.

At the inclusion visit, complete clinical and ophthalmologic retinal examinations were performed in addition to blood and urine sample collection for laboratory analysis. Figure 1 presents the flow chart for designing the experiment.

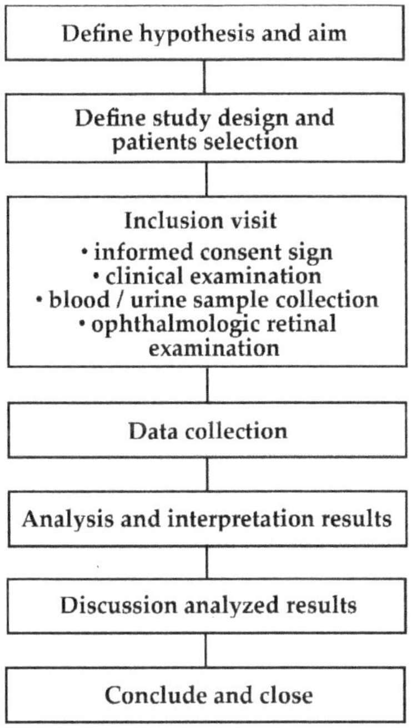

Figure 1. Design of experiment flow chart.

2.3. *Demographic Data and Clinical Characteristics*

The demographic data of patients include age, gender, and diabetes duration. Weight and height were measured using a balance-beam scale and a wall-mounted stadiometer. Body mass index (BMI) was calculated by dividing weight and height squared (kg/m^2) Systolic and diastolic blood pressure were measured by an ambulatory digital sphygmomanometer after a 10 min rest period, and a mean value of three measurements was used.

2.4. *Markers of Glycemic Control and Lipid Metabolism*

Fasting venous blood samples were collected in the morning after an overnight fast to determine metabolic risk factors: hemoglobin A_1c (HbA_{1c}), total cholesterol, HDL cholesterol, LDL cholesterol, and triglycerides. HbA_1c was measured using an automated immunoturbidimetric procedure on a dedicated analyzer (Cobas Integra 400 plus, Roche Ltd., Basel, Switzerland), and serum lipids were determined using standard enzymatic methods on an automated analyzer (Beckman Coulter AU680, Beckman Coulter, Inc., Brea, CA, USA).

2.5. *Indicators of Renal Function*

Renal function was determined using serum creatinine-based glomerular filtration rate (GFR) and albumin-to-creatinine ratio (ACR). Serum creatinine was measured in a fasting blood sample using a routine laboratory method. GFR was estimated using the Chronic Kidney Disease Epidemiology Collaboration (CKD-EPI) formula [20], and a random urine sample was used to determine the ACR by turbidimetric immunoassay and photometric assays. Patients with an ACR < 3 mg/mmol were classified as normoalbuminuric, those with ACR $\geq 3 < 30$ mg/mmol as microalbuminuric, while macroalbuminuria was classified as an ACR $\geq$ 30 mg/mmol. Chronic kidney disease/DN was defined as an estimated GFR < 60 mL/min/1.73 m^2 and/or ACR $\geq$ 30 mg/mmol.

2.6. Ophthalmologic Retinal Examination

The ophthalmologic retinal examination included color fundus photography and optical coherence tomography (OCT) of the macula after mydriasis with eye drops containing 0.5% tropicamide. A conventional 45° fundus camera (Visucam, Zeiss) was used to obtain color fundus images following the EURODIAB (EUROpe and DIABetes) retinal photography methodology [21]. Using the EURODIAB criteria, two retina specialists (M.T., and R.V.) evaluated the images separately, and the final diagnosis for each patient was established based on the DR level of the poorer eye [21]. The macula was examined using Spectral Domain OCT (SD-OCT Copernicus REVO NX, Optopol Technology), and diabetic macular edema (DME) was assessed using the proposed international clinical diabetic retinopathy and diabetic macular edema disease severity ratings [22]. We excluded patients with DME from the study.

2.7. Statistical Analysis

Statistica™ software package version 14.0 (TIBCO Software Inc., Palo Alto, CA, USA) and SPSS software package version 23.0 (IBM, Armonk, NY, USA) were used for statistical analysis. After testing the normality of data distribution using the Kolmogorov–Smirnov test, descriptive results were expressed as means ± SD or median (min-max) for continuous variables and numbers (percentages) for categorical variables. For continuous data, differences between groups were tested by one-way ANOVA and Kruskal–Wallis tests. Scheffe's post-hoc test and multiple comparisons of the Kruskal–Wallis test were used where needed. For categorical data testing, the Chi-square test was used. The Spearman's rank correlation test was used to assess the presence of associations between examined variables. Binary univariate and multiple logistic regression analyses were performed to determine the main predictors of DR, while backward regression analysis was used to detect the main predictors of the ACR. The level of statistical significance was set at 0.05 in all analyses.

3. Results

3.1. Study Population

One hundred and sixty patients with T2DM (96 male/64 female) with a mean age of 64.3 ± 7.6 years and a mean diabetes duration of 14.0 ± 7.1 years were included in this cross-sectional study. Table 1 presents their basic and clinical characteristics, metabolic risk factors, and renal function. Except for elevated mean/median values of BMI (29.8 ± 4.7 kg/m^2), SBP (135 (110–170) mmHg), HbA$_1$c (7.1 (5.5–12.1)%), and LDL cholesterol (2.5 (0.9–7.1) mmol/L), the other analyzed variables—mean/median values of DBP (80 (70–110) mmHg), total cholesterol (4.6 (2.7–10.2) mmol/L), HDL cholesterol (1.3 (0.8–2.5) mmol/L), triglycerides (1.6 (0.5–7.0) mmol/L), serum creatinine (75.5 (42–163) μmol/L), estimated GFR (86.5 (32–108) mL/min/1.73 m^2), and ACR (1.4 (0.3–49.6) mg/mmol)—were within the normal range for patients with T2DM. Corresponding to the medical records, 134 (83.7%) of patients received antihypertensive therapy and 128 (80%) received hypolipemic treatment, of which 108 (67.5%) took statins and 20 (12.5%) took fenofibrate.

According to the level of DR, patients were divided into groups: no DR (n = 86), mild/moderate nonproliferative DR (NPDR) (n = 44), and severe NPDR/proliferative DR (PDR) (n = 30). The three groups did not significantly differ in age, gender, and BMI, but a significant difference was observed in the diabetes duration (p = 0.017), SBP (p = 0.001), DBP (p = 0.003), and HbA$_1$c (p = 0.005) (Table 2). Patients with severe NPDR/PDR had a longer diabetes duration (post-hoc Scheffe test, p = 0.027) and higher SBP (multiple comparisons, p < 0.001) than those with no DR. In contrast, no significant difference in diabetes duration and SBP was observed between the patients with mild/moderate NPDR and those with no DR. Multiple comparisons also showed a significant difference in DBP and HbA$_1$c between the patients with severe NPDR/PDR and those with no DR (DBP, p = 0.017; HbA$_1$c, p = 0.022), as well as patients with mild/moderate NPDR and those with no DR (DBP, $p = 0.043$; HbA_1c, $p = 0.030$). The differences in DBP and HbA_1c between the patients with severe NPDR/PDR and mild/moderate NPDR were not statistically significant. No significant differences in lipids and renal function were found between the groups according to the level of DR.

Table 1. Basic and clinical characteristics, metabolic risk factors, and renal function of all patients with type 2 diabetes ($n = 160$) included in the study.

	All Patients Included in the Study ($n = 160$)
Age (years)	64.3 ± 7.6
Gender (m/f) (%)	60/40
Diabetes duration (years)	14.0 ± 7.1
BMI (kg/m^2)	29.8 ± 4.7
SBP (mmHg)	135 (110–170)
DBP (mmHg)	80 (70–110)
HbA_1c (%)	7.1 (5.5–12.1)
Total cholesterol (mmol/L)	4.6 (2.7–10.2)
HDL cholesterol (mmol/L)	1.3 (0.8–2.5)
LDL cholesterol (mmol/L)	2.5 (0.9–7.1)
Triglycerides (mmol/L)	1.6 (0.5–7.0)
Serum creatinine (μmol/L)	75.5 (42–163)
ACR (mg/mmol)	1.4 (0.3–49.6)
eGFR (mL/min/1.73 m^2)	86.5 (32–108)

Legend: Values are means ± SD, percentages, or medians (min-max). BMI indicates body mass index; SBP: systolic blood pressure; DBP: diastolic blood pressure; HbA_1c: glycated hemoglobin; HDL: high-density lipoprotein cholesterol; LDL: low-density lipoprotein cholesterol; eGFR: estimated glomerular filtration rate; ACR: albumin-to-creatinine ratio.

Table 2. Diabetes duration, systolic and diastolic blood pressure, and HbA_1c of patients with type 2 diabetes ($n = 160$). Patients were divided into three groups according to the level of diabetic retinopathy.

	No DR ($n = 86$)	**Mild/Moderate NPDR ($n = 44$)**	**Severe NPDR/PDR ($n = 30$)**	***p*-Value**
Diabetes duration	11.98 ± 6.76	15.60 ± 8.23	16.91 ± 5.88	0.017
SBP (mmHg)	130 (115–170)	137 (110–170)	150 (120–170)	0.001
DBP (mmHg)	80 (70–95)	85 (70–110)	85 (75–100)	0.003
HbA_1c (%)	6.7 (5.5–9.4)	7.3 (5.8–9.2)	7.8 (5.6–12.1)	0.005

Legend: Values are means ± SD or medians (min-max). SBP indicates systolic blood pressure; DBP: diastolic blood pressure; HbA_1c: glycated hemoglobin; DR: diabetic retinopathy; NPDR: nonproliferative diabetic retinopathy; NPDR/PDR: nonproliferative diabetic retinopathy/proliferative diabetic retinopathy.

3.2. Prevalence of Microvascular Complications and Their Correlations

In our study cohort, the prevalence of DR was 46.3%. Of the 74 with DR, 44 (59.5%) had mild or moderate NPDR, and 30 (40.5%) had severe NPDR or PDR.

The prevalence of DN according to the eGFR category was 32.6%, though its prevalence according to the ACR classification was 12.5%. Of the 92 with eGFR $\leq$ 90 mL/min/1.73 m^2, 62 (67.4%) had eGFR 60–89 mL/min/1.73 m^2, while 30 (32.6%) had eGFR $\leq$ 59 mL/min/1.73 m^2. Of the 32 with an ACR higher than 3 mg/mmol, an ACR of 3–30 mg/mmol was found in 28 (87.5%) patients, and an ACR > 30 mg/mmol only in 4 (12.5%) of them.

DR was positively associated with diabetes duration ($R = 0.276454$, $p = 0.013$), HbA_1c ($R = 0.361563$, $p < 0.001$), SBP ($R = 0.465979$, $p < 0.001$), and DBP ($R = 0.379747$, $p < 0.001$) (Figure 2A–D). No significant correlation was observed between DR and age, BMI, serum lipids, and renal function ($p > 0.05$).

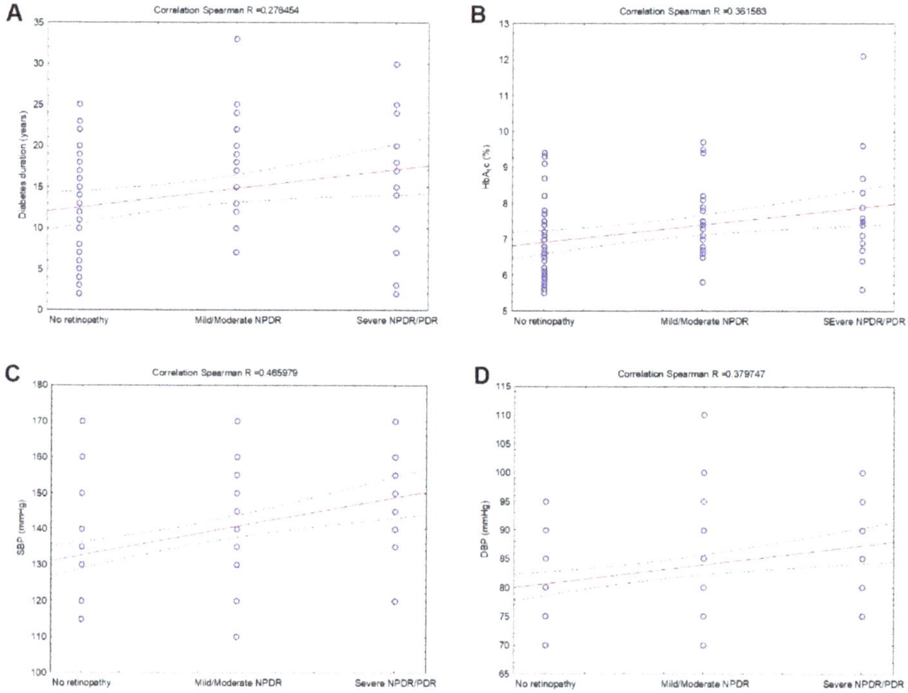

Figure 2. Correlations between diabetic retinopathy, diabetes duration (**A**), HbA_1c (**B**), systolic blood pressure (SBP) (**C**), and diastolic blood pressure (DBP) (**D**) in patients with T2DM included in the study. Legend of the correlation linear scatterplot: blue circles—plots (means or medians); red solid line—linear correlation line; red dotted lines—0.95 confidence interval.

ACR was positively related to diabetes duration (R = 0.241504, $p = 0.034$) and HbA_1c (R = 0.231647, $p = 0.043$) (Figure 3A,B). No significant relation was observed between the ACR and age, BMI, serum lipids, SBP, and DBP ($p > 0.05$). Estimated GFR was negatively related only to age (R = −0.544649, $p < 0.001$), but no significant relation was found between eGFR and other analyzed variables.

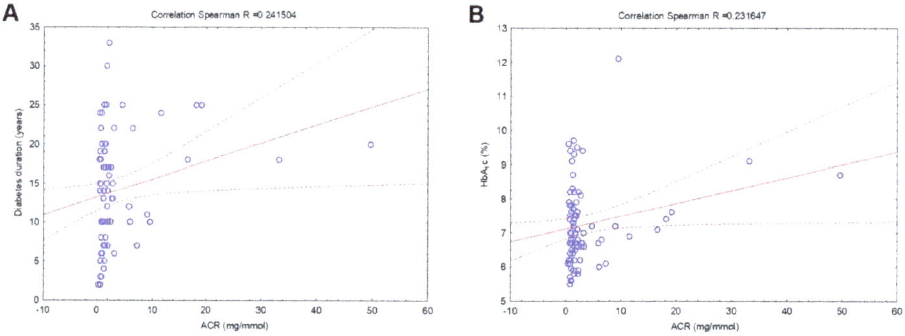

Figure 3. Correlations between the albumin-to-creatinine ratio (ACR ratio), diabetes duration (**A**), and HbA_1c (**B**) in patients with T2DM included in the study. Legend of the correlation linear scatterplot: blue circles—plots (means or medians); red solid line—linear correlation line; red dotted lines—0.95 confidence interval.

3.3. Predictors of Diabetic Retinopathy and Nephropathy

Binary logistic regression analysis (no DR/DR) showed that longer diabetes duration ($p = 0.008$), poor glycemic control (HbA_1c) ($p = 0.008$), higher SBP ($p = 0.001$), and DBP ($p = 0.003$) were the main predictors of DR. However, even after adjustment for diabetes duration and HbA_1c, there were significant effects of SBP (AOR = 1.06, $p = 0.004$) and DBP (AOR = 1.12, $p = 0.007$) on DR development (Table 3). No significant relation between DR and other analyzed variables using logistic regression analysis was observed.

Table 3. Results of logistic regression analysis for diabetic retinopathy in patients with type 2 diabetes as a dichotomous dependent variable.

Variable	OR (95% CI)	*p*-Value	AOR (95% CI) *	*p*-Value *
Diabetes duration	1.10 (1.02–1.18)	0.008	/	
HbA_1c	1.87 (1.17–2.99)	0.008	/	
SBP	1.07 (1.03–1.11)	0.001	1.06 (1.02–1.11)	0.004
DBP	1.12 (1.04–1.21)	0.003	1.12 (1.03–1.22)	0.007

* OR after adjustment for diabetes duration and HbA_1c. Legend: HbA_1c indicates glycated hemoglobin; SBP: systolic blood pressure; DBP: diastolic blood pressure.

The results of backward regression analysis for ACR as a dependent variable are presented in Table 4, and those for eGFR as a dependent variable are in Table 5. The best model for predicting ACR ($R^2 = 0.258$) obtained by backward regression included only a longer diabetes duration ($p = 0.034$), while the best model for predicting eGFR ($R^2 = 0.307$) involved only age ($p < 0.001$).

Table 4. Results of backward regression analysis for albumin-to-creatinine ratio in patients with type 2 diabetes as a dependent variable.

	Unstandardized Coefficients		Standardized Coefficients		
Model	**B**	**Std. Error**	**Beta**	**t**	**Sig.**
(Constant)	0.138	1.839		0.075	0.941
Diabetes duration	0.252	0.117	0.242	2.155	0.034

Dependent variable: albumin-to-creatinine ratio. $R^2 = 0.258$.

Table 5. Results of backward regression analysis for estimated glomerular filtration rate in patients with type 2 diabetes as a dependent variable.

	Unstandardized Coefficients		Standardized Coefficients		
Model	**B**	**Std. Error**	**Beta**	**t**	**Sig.**
(Constant)	0.138	1.839		0.075	0.941
Age	−1.413	0.247	−0.554	−5.728	<0.001

Dependent variable: estimated glomerular filtration rate. $R^2 = 0.307$.

4. Discussion

The results of our study suggest that SBP and DBP are independent risk factors for DR in patients with T2DM. Less than half of the studied patients with T2DM had DR (46.3%), and most patients had satisfactory glucose control (HbA_1c 7.1%). Although DR and DN are essential microvascular complications connected with a similar pathogenesis and often coincide, there were no associations between DR and renal function measured with eGFR and ACR. However, the prevalence of DN in our study, defined as an ACR $\geq$ 30 mg/mmol and estimated GFR < 60 mL/min/1.73 m^2, was moderate to relatively high (12.5% and 32.6%). Also, no associations existed between DR and age, BMI, and serum lipids. Finally, binary logistic regression analysis (no DR/DR) showed that longer diabetes duration

(p = 0.008), poor glycemic control (HbA_1c) (p = 0.008), higher SBP (p = 0.001), and DBP (p = 0.003) were the main risk factors of DR. However, even after adjustment for diabetes duration and HbA_1c, SBP (AOR = 1.06, p = 0.004) and DBP (AOR = 1.12, p = 0.007) had significant effects on DR development.

The epidemiological studies confirmed the connection between high blood pressure and DR and showed that blood pressure is not only a risk factor for DR because the treatment of hypertension is beneficial [23]. Large, prospective trials that included patients with T2DM, like ABCD (Appropriate Blood Pressure Control in Diabetes) and UKPDS (The UK Prospective Diabetes Study), suggest that strict blood pressure control can prevent the development and progression of DR [24,25]. Patients with T2DM and SBP $\geq$ 140 mmHg have a 2.8 times higher risk of developing DR than those with SBP < 125 mmHg [23]. In addition, in those with borderline increased blood pressure (up to 144/82 mmHg), a 35% risk reduction in DR progression and photocoagulation can be achieved with a decrease in SBP by 10 mmHg and with a reduction in DBP by 5 mmHg. In our study, the patients had even lower median systolic and diastolic blood pressure (135/80 mmHg). The Steno 2 study included patients with T2DM and microalbuminuria and found a 55% lower risk of DR progression according to the EURODIAB scale with the intensive control of hypertension [26]. Irrespective of normal or high blood pressure, SBP is significantly related to the DR presence in patients with T2DM, even after adjusting for the duration of diabetes, gender, and HbA_1c [17]. SBP is also associated with incipient and advanced DR independently of the presence of cardiovascular and renal disease [27]. Besides blood pressure level, its variability is also a risk factor for DR in patients with T2DM [28]. Most studies found a link between DR and SBP, but some researchers discovered that only DBP relates to DR [29]. Contrarily, a randomized controlled ADVANCE trial showed that blood pressure control within the normal range (below 140/80 mm Hg) had no effect in preventing DR progression [30].

Hypertension, pregnancy, autonomic neuropathy, and hyperglycemia increase retinal blood flow and lead to a progression of DR, while normoglycemia and the moderate stenosis of the carotid artery decrease retinal blood flow and have a protective effect on DR [31–35]. Retinal blood flow distribution is regulated by central mechanisms controlled by autonomic innervation and local mechanisms through autoregulation. The impaired autoregulation in patients with T2DM potentiated with hyperglycemia significantly increases blood flow and mean arterial pressure, established a vicious circle between retinal hemodynamic changes, hyperglycemia, and hypertension [32]. Several other conditions are implicated in impaired autoregulation in patients with T2DM, like the reduced contractile capability of retinal pericytes, capillary basement thickening, and arteriolar hyalinosis, resulting in the direct transmission of increased blood pressure to the retinal microvasculature [33]. According to studies, hypertension can also cause oxidative stress and inflammation [36]. It appears that the coexistence of hyperglycemia and hypertension can aggravate inflammation and oxidative stress, both of which are pathogenic processes implicated in the development and progression of DR.

Increased blood pressure has a role in the pathological changes of DR, participates in the local renin–angiotensin system (RAS), and may damage retinal capillary endothelial cells [27,37]. Although the exact mechanism of high blood pressure damage in patients with DR is not fully understood, it is well known that chronic hyperglycemia via endothelial dysfunction aggravates the blood–retinal barrier, resulting in impaired retinal perfusion [38–40]. High blood pressure upregulates vascular endothelial growth factor (VEGF), a potent angiogenic factor and essential growth factor for vascular endothelial cells, which has a vital role in the presence and severity of DR. In addition, an increase in angiotensin-II, observed in patients with hypertension, results in its binding to the AT-I receptor that also upregulates the VEGF [41]. Finally, VEGF induces essential changes related to DR development and progression, like basement membrane thickening, increased vascular permeability, and neovascularization [42] (Figure 4).

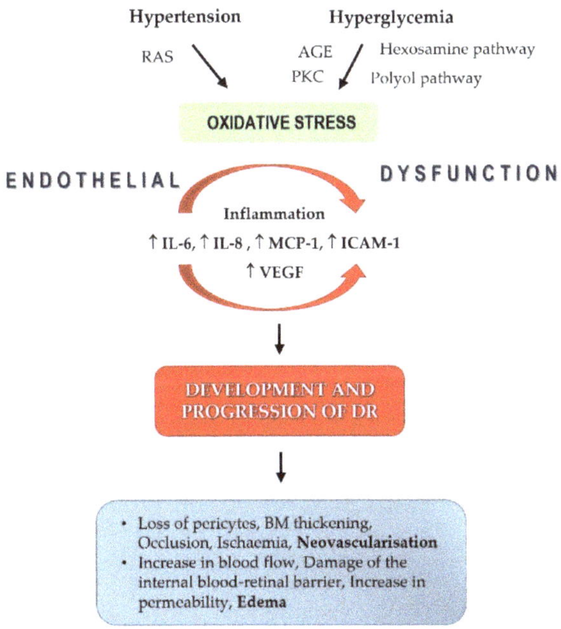

Figure 4. Risk factors for diabetic retinopathy development and progression mentioned in the Discussion.

Although blood pressure control has protective effects on DR development and progression, the question is which blood pressure value is optimal for patients with DR. It seems that targeting very low systolic and diastolic blood pressure (below 120/80 mmHg) has no additional beneficial effects [43]. A combination of optimal blood pressure control (SBP below 140 mmHg) and glucose control (HbA_{1C} below 7.0%) significantly reduces the probability of DR presence in patients with T2DM [44]. Normotensive patients with T2DM must be screened for DR because about 20% of them have DR, and in those patients, an increase in SBP is independently and significantly associated with DR development and progression [17]. RAS inhibitors should be introduced after diagnosing hypertension in patients with T2DM and DR because of their possible beneficial effects on DR. RAS inhibitors not only decrease the risk of development and progression of DR but also increase the possibility of DR regression, which is suggested in a meta-analysis that included 21 randomized clinical trials with 13,823 participants. Also, ACE inhibitors might be better than angiotensin-receptor blockers in treating DR and are the drug of choice for those with DR [45].

Although the prevalence of DN according to the eGFR category in our study was relatively high (32.6%), DR was not associated with eGFR and ACR. Previous studies observed a significant connection between DR and DN and proposed that DN precedes DR in patients with T2DM [46]. High blood glucose, high systolic and diastolic blood pressure, and duration of disease simultaneously connect the parallel development of DR and DN. However, DR is present and may progress in about 30% of patients with type 1 diabetes and strictly normal renal function (normoalbuminuria and eGFR over 60 mL/min/1.73 m^2) [19]. In addition, many patients with T2DM and renal abnormalities (proteinuria and/or renal insufficiency) showed no signs of DR [11].

In our study, no significant relation was obtained between the ACR and age, BMI, serum lipids, SBP, and DBP. Although dyslipidemia is related to the pathogenesis of DN, discordant associations of lipid parameters with albuminuria were found [47]. Also, obesity is generally associated with increased ACR, although severe obesity compared with milder obesity status cannot predict the occurrence of increased ACR and microalbuminuria [48]. It is well known that the prevalence of chronic kidney disease and albuminuria rises with age, although recent epidemiological studies suggest that the albuminuria-associated risk of all-cause mortality and cardiovascular mortality is attenuated in elderly patients with diabetes [49]. In addition, the interaction between albuminuria stages and age groups was not significant in elderly individuals of various ages with diabetes [50].

The present study and results have several potential limitations. First, our study was cross-sectional and included a limited number of patients with T2DM. Therefore, the data must be confirmed in prospective studies with more patients. Second, we used a single-office blood pressure measurement that cannot rule out hypertension in patients with diabetes, for which ambulatory blood pressure can provide an excellent prognostic benefit [51]. The procedure used in our study to diagnose the presence and severity of DR and previously described blood-pressure-measurement deficiency may influence the final results, making it difficult to compare findings between studies. Third, since our study included only the white European population, there was no racial/ethnic diversity. Fourth, a small number of DR predictors is also a study limitation.

In conclusion, the results of our study suggest that systolic and diastolic blood pressure are independent risk factors for DR in patients with T2DM with and without DN. The study was conducted on patients with satisfactory glucose control with T2DM. The result of the study implies that we should regularly monitor blood pressure in patients with T2DM, even in those without hypertension and with optimal glucose control, to prevent the development of DR.

Author Contributions: Conceptualization, T.B. and M.T.; data curation, M.T.; formal analysis, T.B. and M.T.; methodology, T.B., M.T., R.V., N.B. and S.L.; project administration, T.B. and S.L.; resources, T.B., supervision, N.B. and S.L.; writing—Original draft, T.B. and M.T.; writing—Review and editing, T.B., M.T., R.V., N.B. and S.L. All authors have read and agreed to the published version of the manuscript.

Funding: This research received no specific grant from any funding agency in the public, commercial, or not-for-profit sectors.

Institutional Review Board Statement: The research was conducted after consideration and approval by a Hospital's Ethics Committee (protocol number 05/01-849, approval date: 16 September 2020) following the Declaration of Helsinki.

Informed Consent Statement: Before any procedures and inclusion in the study, patients received written and oral information about the study and signed informed consent.

Data Availability Statement: The data presented in this study are available on request from the corresponding author.

Conflicts of Interest: The authors declare no conflict of interest.

References

1. Saeedi, P.; Petersohn, I.; Salpea, P.; Malanda, B.; Karuranga, S.; Unwin, N.; Colagiuri, S.; Guariguata, L.; Motala, A.A.; Ogurtsova, K.; et al. Global and regional diabetes prevalence estimates for 2019 and projections for 2030 and 2045: Results from the International Diabetes Federation Diabetes Atlas, 9th edition. *Diabetes Res. Clin. Pract.* **2019**, *157*, 107843. [CrossRef] [PubMed]
2. Tomic, D.; Shaw, J.E.; Magliano, D.J. The burden and risks of emerging complications of diabetes mellitus. *Nat. Rev. Endocrinol.* **2022**, *18*, 525–539. [CrossRef] [PubMed]
3. Van Hecke, M.V.; Dekker, J.M.; Stehouwer, C.D.; Polak, B.C.; Fuller, J.H.; Sjolie, A.K.; Kofinis, A.; Rottiers, R.; Porta, M.; Chaturvedi, N. EURODIAB prospective complications study. Diabetic retinopathy is associated with mortality and cardiovascular disease incidence: The EURODIAB Prospective Complications Study. *Diabetes Care* **2005**, *28*, 1383–1389. [CrossRef] [PubMed]
4. Yau, J.W.; Rogers, S.L.; Kawasaki, R.; Lamoureux, E.L.; Kowalski, J.W.; Bek, T. Global prevalence and major risk factors of diabetic retinopathy. *Diabetes Care* **2012**, *35*, 556–564. [CrossRef]
5. Klein, R.; Klein, B.E.K. Blood pressure control and diabetic retinopathy. *Br. J. Ophthalmol.* **2002**, *86*, 365–367. [CrossRef]
6. Shaya, F.T.; Aljawadi, M. Diabetic retinopathy. *Clin. Ophthalmol.* **2007**, *1*, 259–265.
7. Poulsen, P.L.; Bek, T.; Ebbehøj, E.; Hansen, K.W.; Mogensen, C.E. 24-h ambulatory blood pressure and retinopathy in normoalbuminuric IDDM patients. *Diabetologia* **1998**, *41*, 105–110. [CrossRef]

8. Mbata, O.; Abo El-Magd, N.F.; El-Remessy, A.B. Obesity, metabolic syndrome and diabetic retinopathy: Beyond hyperglycemia. *World. J. Diabetes* **2017**, *15*, 317–329. [CrossRef]
9. Grunwald, J.E.; Alexander, J.; Ying, G.S.; Maguire, M.; Daniel, E.; Whittock-Martin, R.; Parker, C.; McWilliams, K.; Lo, J.C.; Go, A.; et al. Retinopathy and chronic kidney disease in the Chronic Renal Insufficiency Cohort (CRIC) study. *Arch. Ophthalmol.* **2012**, *130*, 1136–1144. [CrossRef]
10. Arar, N.H.; Freedman, B.I.; Adler, S.G.; Iyengar, S.K.; Chew, E.Y.; Davis, M.D.; Satko, S.G.; Bowden, D.W.; Duggirala, R.; Elston, R.C.; et al. Heritability of the severity of diabetic retinopathy: The FIND-eye study. *Inv. Ophthalmol. Vis. Sci.* **2008**, *9*, 3839–3844. [CrossRef]
11. Wolf, G.; Müller, N.; Mandecka, A.; Müller, U.A. Association of diabetic retinopathy and renal function in patients with types 1 and 2 diabetes mellitus. *Clin. Nephrol.* **2007**, *68*, 81–86. [CrossRef]
12. Tolonen, N.; Hietala, K.; Forsblom, C.; Harjutsalo, V.; Makinen, V.P.; Kyto, J.; Summanen, P.A.; Thorn, L.M.; Wadén, J.; Gordin, D.; et al. Associations and interactions between lipid profiles, retinopathy and nephropathy in patients with type 1 diabetes: The FinnDiane Study. *J. Intern. Med.* **2013**, *274*, 469–479. [CrossRef] [PubMed]
13. Li, Y.; Su, X.; Ye, Q.; Guo, X.; Xu, B.; Guan, T.; Chen, A. The predictive value of diabetic retinopathy on subsequent diabetic nephropathy in patients with type 2 diabetes: A systematic review and meta-analysis of prospective studies. *Ren. Fail.* **2021**, *43*, 231–240. [CrossRef] [PubMed]
14. Kohner, E.M. Diabetic retinopathy. *Br. Med. Bull.* **1989**, *45*, 148–173. [CrossRef] [PubMed]
15. Stratton, I.M.; Kohner, E.M.; Aldington, S.J.; Turner, R.C.; Holman, R.R.; Manley, S.E.; Matthews, D.R. UKPDS 50: Risk factors for incidence and progression of retinopathy in type II diabetes over 6 years from diagnosis. *Diabetologia* **2001**, *44*, 156–163. [CrossRef]
16. Emdin, C.A.; Rahimi, K.; Neal, B.; Callender, T.; Perkovic, V.; Patel, A. Blood pressure lowering in type 2 diabetes: A systematic review and meta-analysis. *JAMA* **2015**, *313*, 603–615. [CrossRef] [PubMed]
17. Li, Y.T.; Wang, Y.; Hu, X.Y.; Chen, J.H.; Li, Y.Y.; Zhong, Q.Y.; Cheng, H.; Mohammed, B.H.; Liang, X.L.; Hernandez, J.; et al. Association between Systolic Blood Pressure and Diabetic Retinopathy in Both Hypertensive and Normotensive Patients with Type 2 Diabetes: Risk Factors and Healthcare Implications. *Healthcare* **2021**, *9*, 580. [CrossRef] [PubMed]
18. Tomić, M.; Vrabec, R.; Ljubić, S.; Bulum, T.; Prkačin, I.; Rahelić, D. Renal function is associated with cataract development in patients with type 2 diabetes. *Acta. Clin. Croat.* **2021**, *60* (Suppl. S1), 18–23. [CrossRef]
19. Bulum, T.; Blaslov, K.; Duvnjak, L. Risk factors for development and progression of nonproliferative retinopathy in normoalbuminuric patients with type 1 diabetes. *Diabetes Res. Clin. Pract.* **2014**, *106*, 555–559. [CrossRef]
20. Levey, A.S.; Stevens, L.A. Estimating GFR using the CKD Epidemiology Collaboration (CKD-EPI) creatinine equation: More accurate GFR estimates, lower CKD prevalence estimates, and better risk predictions. *Am. J. Kidney Dis.* **2010**, *55*, 622–627. [CrossRef]
21. Aldington, S.J.; Kohner, E.M.; Meuer, S.; Klein, R.; Sjølie, A.K. Methodology for retinal photography and assessment of diabetic retinopathy: The EURODIAB IDDM complications study. *Diabetologia* **1995**, *38*, 437–444. [CrossRef] [PubMed]
22. Wilkinson, C.P.; Ferris, F.L., 3rd; Klein, R.E.; Lee, P.P.; Agardh, C.D.; Davis, M.; Dills, D.; Kampik, A.; Pararajasegaram, R.; Verdaguer, J.T. Proposed international clinical diabetic retinopathy and diabetic macular edema disease severity scales. *Ophthalmology* **2003**, *110*, 1677–1682. [CrossRef]
23. Gillow, J.T.; Gibson, J.M.; Dodson, P.M. Hypertension and diabetic retinopathy-what's the story? *Br. J. Ophthalmol.* **1999**, *83*, 1083–1087. [CrossRef] [PubMed]
24. Matthews, D.R.; Stratton, I.M.; Aldington, S.; Holman, R.R.; Kohner, E.M.; UK Prospective Diabetes Study Group. Risks of progression of retinopathy and vision loss related to tight blood pressure control in type 2 diabetes mellitus (UKPDS 69). *Arch. Ophthalmol.* **2004**, *122*, 1631–1640. [CrossRef] [PubMed]
25. Schrier, R.W.; Estacio, R.O.; Mehler, P.S.; Hiattet, W.R. Appropriate blood pressure control in hypertensive and normotensive type 2 diabetes mellitus: A summary of the ABCD trial. *Nat. Clin. Pract. Nephrol.* **2007**, *3*, 428–438. [CrossRef] [PubMed]
26. Gaede, P.; Vedel, P.; Parving, H.; Pedersenet, O. Intensified multifactorial intervention in patients with type 2 diabetes and microalbuminuria: The Steno type 2 randomized study. *Lancet* **1999**, *353*, 617–622. [CrossRef]
27. Liu, L.; Quang, N.D.; Banu, R.; Kumar, H.; Tham, Y.-C.; Cheng, C.-Y.; Wong, T.Y.; Sabanayagam, C. Hypertension, blood pressure control and diabetic retinopathy in a large population-based study. *PLoS ONE* **2020**, *15*, e0229665. [CrossRef]
28. Lou, Q.; Chen, X.; Wang, K.; Liu, H.; Zhang, Z.; Lee, Y. The Impact of Systolic Blood Pressure, Pulse Pressure, and Their Variability on Diabetes Retinopathy among Patients with Type 2 Diabetes. *J. Diabetes Res.* **2022**, *2022*, 7876786. [CrossRef]
29. Rajalakshmi, R.; Amutha, A.; Ranjani, H.; Ali, M.K.; Unnikrishnan, R.; Anjana, R.M.; Narayan, K.M.V.; Mohan, V. Prevalence and risk factors for diabetic retinopathy in Asian Indians with young onset type 1 and type 2 diabetes. *J. Diabetes Complicat.* **2014**, *28*, 291–297. [CrossRef]
30. Patel, A.; MacMahon, S.; Chalmers, J.; Neal, B.; Woodward, M.; Billot, L.; Harrap, S.; Poulter, N.; Marre, M.; Cooper, M.; et al. Effects of a fixed combination of perindopril and indapamide on macrovascular and microvascular outcomes in patients with type 2 diabetes mellitus (the ADVANCE trial): A randomised controlled trial. *Lancet* **2007**, *370*, 829–840. [CrossRef]
31. Kohner, E.M.; Patel, V.; Rassam, S.M.B. Role of blood flow and impaired auto-regulation in the pathogenesis of diabetic retinopathy. *Diabetes* **1995**, *44*, 603–607. [CrossRef]
32. Grunwald, J.E.; Dupont, J.; Riva, C.E. Retinal haemodynamics in patients with early diabetes mellitus. *Br. J. Ophthalmol.* **1996**, *80*, 327–331. [CrossRef] [PubMed]

33. Fuchsjäger-Mayrl, G.; Polak, K.; Luksch, A.; Polska, E.; Dorner, G.T.; Rainer, G.; Eichler, H.G.; Schmetterer, L. Retinal blood flow and systemic blood pressure in healthy young subjects. *Graefes. Arch. Clin. Exp. Ophthalmol.* **2001**, *239*, 673–677. [CrossRef] [PubMed]
34. Pota, C.E.; Apaydın, K.C. Retinal and choroidal microvascular changes during pregnancy detected with OCTA. *Can. J. Ophthalmol.* 2023, *in press*. [CrossRef]
35. István, L.; Czakó, C.; Benyó, F.; Élő, A.; Mihály, Z.; Sótonyi, P.; Varga, A.; Nagy, Z.Z.; Kovács, I. The effect of systemic factors on retinal blood flow in patients with carotid stenosis: An optical coherence tomography angiography study. *Geroscience* **2022**, *44*, 389–401. [CrossRef]
36. Vaziri, N.D.; Rodriguez-Iturbe, B. Mechanisms of disease: Oxidative stress and inflammation in the pathogenesis of hypertension. *Nat. Clin. Pract. Nephrol.* **2006**, *2*, 582–593. [CrossRef] [PubMed]
37. Sjølie, A.K.; Dodsonand, P.; Hobbs, F.R.R. Does renin-angiotensin system blockade have a role in preventing diabetic retinopathy? A clinical review. *Int. J. Clin. Pract.* **2011**, *65*, 148–153. [CrossRef]
38. Cardoso, C.R.L.; Leite, N.C.; Dib, E.; Salles, G.F. Predictors of development and progression of retinopathy in patients with type 2 diabetes: Importance of blood pressure parameters. *Sci. Rep.* **2017**, *7*, 4867. [CrossRef]
39. Do, D.V.; Wang, X.; Vedula, S.S.; Marrone, M.; Sleilati, G.; Hawkins, B.S.; Frank, R.N. Blood pressure control for diabetic retinopathy. *Cochrane. Database. Syst. Rev.* **2015**, *1*, CD006127. [CrossRef]
40. Fraser-Bell, S.; Symes, R.; Vaze, A. Hypertensive eye disease: A review. *Clin. Exp. Ophthalmol.* **2017**, *45*, 45–53. [CrossRef]
41. Schlingerman, R.O.; Hinsbergh, V.W.M. Role of vascular permeability factor/vascular endothelial growth factor in eye disease. *Br. J. Ophthalmol.* **1997**, *81*, 501–502. [CrossRef] [PubMed]
42. Apte, R.S.; Chen, D.S.; Ferrara, N. VEGF in Signaling and Disease: Beyond Discovery and Development. *Cell* **2019**, *176*, 1248–1264. [CrossRef] [PubMed]
43. Hansson, L.; Zanchetti, A.; Carruthers, S.G. Effects of intensive blood pressure lowering and low dose aspirin in patients with hypertension: Principal results of the hypertension optimal treatment (HOT) randomized trial. *Lancet* **1998**, *351*, 1755–1762. [CrossRef]
44. Pan, C.-W.; Wang, S.; Xu, C.-L.; Song, E. Combined effect of glycemic and blood pressure control on diabetic retinopathy among Chinese with type-2 diabetes mellitus. *Diabetol. Metab. Syndr.* **2018**, *10*, 73. [CrossRef]
45. Wang, B.; Wang, F.; Zhang, Y.; Zhao, S.-H.; Zhao, W.-J.; Yan, S.-L.; Wang, Y.-G. Effects of RAS inhibitors on diabetic retinopathy: A systematic review and meta-analysis. *Lancet Diabetes Endocrinol.* **2015**, *3*, 263–274. [CrossRef] [PubMed]
46. Kotlarsky, P.; Bolotin, A.; Dorfman, K.; Knyazer, B.; Lifshitz, T.; Levy, J. Link between retinopathy and nephropathy caused by complications of diabetes mellitus type 2. *Int. Ophthalmol.* **2015**, *35*, 59–66. [CrossRef]
47. Sun, K.; Lin, D.; Li, F.; Huang, C.; Qi, Y.; Xue, S.; Tang, J.; Yang, C.; Li, Y.; Ren, M.; et al. Discordant associations of lipid parameters with albuminuria and chronic kidney disease: A population-based study. *Lipids Health Dis.* **2015**, *14*, 152. [CrossRef]
48. Minoo, F.; Mahdavi-Mazdeh, M.; Abbasi, M.R.; Sohrabi, S. Impact of the severity of obesity on microalbuminuria in obese normotensive nondiabetic individuals. *J. Renal. Inj. Prev.* **2015**, *4*, 34–38. [CrossRef]
49. Tancredi, M.; Rosengren, A.; Svensson, A.M.; Kosiborod, M.; Pivodic, A.; Gudbjörnsdottir, S.; Wedel, H.; Clements, M.; Dahlqvist, S.; Lind, M. Excess Mortality among Persons with Type 2 Diabetes. *N. Engl. J. Med.* **2015**, *373*, 1720–1732. [CrossRef]
50. Hwang, S.; Lee, K.; Park, J.; Kim, D.H.; Jeon, J.; Jang, H.R.; Hur, K.Y.; Kim, J.H.; Huh, W.; Kim, Y.G.; et al. Prognostic significance of albuminuria in elderly of various ages with diabetes. *Sci. Rep.* **2023**, *13*, 7079. [CrossRef]
51. Gupta, H.; Vidhale, T.; Pustake, M.; Gandhi, C.; Roy, T. Utility of ambulatory blood pressure monitoring in detection of masked hypertension and risk of hypertension mediated organ damage in normotensive patients with type 2 diabetes mellitus. *Blood Press.* **2022**, *31*, 50–57. [CrossRef] [PubMed]

biomedicines

MDPI

Article

Prediabetes, Non-Dipping Profile and Hypertension—A Recipe for Increased Arterial Stiffness

Juraj Jug [1,2], Điđi Delalić [2], Valerija Bralić Lang [2,3], Tomislav Bulum [2,4,*] and Ingrid Prkačin [2,5]

1 Health Center Zagreb-West, 10000 Zagreb, Croatia
2 School of Medicine, University of Zagreb, 10000 Zagreb, Croatia
3 Family medicine practice Valerija Bralić Lang, 10000 Zagreb, Croatia
4 Vuk Vrhovac University Clinic for Diabetes, Endocrinology and Metabolic Diseases, Merkur University Hospital, 10000 Zagreb, Croatia
5 Department of Internal E.R., Merkur University Hospital, 10000 Zagreb, Croatia
* Correspondence: tomobulum@gmail.com; Tel.: +385-1-235-3887; Fax: +385-1-233-1515

Abstract: Background: Pulse wave velocity (PWV) is a known predictor of target organ damage, cardiovascular disease and overall mortality. The aim of this study was to compare the PWV values in subjects with prediabetes, a non-dipper profile and arterial hypertension with their values in healthy subjects. Methods: A total of 301 subjects, aged 40–70 years, without diabetes mellitus were included in this cross-sectional study (150 with prediabetes). They underwent a 24 h ambulatory blood pressure monitoring (ABPM). Subjects were divided into three hypertension groups (A = healthy, B = controlled hypertension, C = uncontrolled hypertension). Dipping status was determined according to ABPM results, and PWV was measured by an oscillometric device. Prediabetes was defined as having 2 separate fasting plasma glucose (FPG) measurements between 5.6 and 6.9 mmol/L. Results: The highest PWV values were found in group C (9.60 ± 1.34 vs. 8.46 ± 1.01 in group B vs. 7.79 ± 1.10 in group A; $p < 0.001$), in subjects with prediabetes (8.98 ± 1.31 m/s vs. 8.26 ± 1.22 m/s; $p < 0.001$) and in prediabetic non-dippers among age groups ($p = 0.05$). In the multivariate regression model age, blood pressure, nocturnal indices and FPG were shown as independent predictors of PWV values. Conclusion: Significantly higher PWV values were found in subjects with prediabetes and non-dipping profiles in all three examined hypertension groups.

Keywords: arterial stiffness; blood pressure; hypertension; prediabetes; pulse wave velocity; target organ damage

1. Introduction

Prediabetes (PreD) is a heterogeneous condition of impaired glucose metabolism in which the values do not meet the criteria for type 2 diabetes mellitus (T2DM) but are higher t the values considered normal. To have PreD, it is necessary to meet one or more set of criteria in at least two separate laboratory measurements (American Diabetes Association, ADA, 2017): fasting plasma glucose (FPG) 5.6–6.9 mmol/L, or HbA1c 5.7–6.4%, or blood glucose values by oral glucose load test 75 g glucose (OGTT) after 2 h 7.8–11.0 mmol/L [1]. Similarly, the guidelines of the European Society of Cardiology (ESC), in collaboration with the European Association for the Study of Diabetes (EASD), differ only in concentrations of FPG in which those of 6.1–6.9 mmol/L represent PreD. They both agree that testing is required in all persons over 45 years of age, and at any age if there is a high risk of developing prediabetes (BMI > 25 kg/m^2, first-degree relative with diabetes, women who were diagnosed with gestational diabetes mellitus, hypertension, polycystic ovary syndrome, etc.) [1,2].

PreD is associated with a 20% higher risk of cardiovascular disease (CVD), especially carotid atherosclerosis and coronary artery calcification, while the association declines with aging, probably as a result of the influence of other risk factors [3–5]. Although some studies suggested that dietary or exercise interventions can prevent CVD in people with PreD, the risk should still be minimized by removing other risk factors for the development of CVD that are almost identical to those for the development of PreD [3].

Micro- and macrovascular damage are associated with PreD and are presented by greater arterial stiffness and faster progression of atherosclerosis. The gold standard for determining arterial stiffness is pulse wave velocity (PWV) using tonometry or oscillometric devices; arterial stiffness is a known predictor of target organ damage (TOD), CVD and overall mortality [6–8]. An increase in PWV of 1 m/s compared to the reference value for age and sex is associated with a 14% higher cardiovascular (CV) risk [9,10]. Notably, PWV values are physiologically higher in women in all age groups [11]. A study from Loehr et al. [12] on cohort members of the Atherosclerosis Risk in Communities (ARIC) study (4682 participants), demonstrated a significant association of PreD with brachial PWV. It is also known that hyperglycemia with hyperinsulinemia acutely increases PWV, heart rate and diastolic blood pressure (DBP) in healthy people, possibly due to an increase in sympathetic tone [13]. Reduction of PWV can be achieved by good control of arterial hypertension (AH) and other risk factors, thus reducing CV and mortality [14].

The absence of a drop in BP at night (non-dipping profile) is also a significant risk factor in the development of CVD, and it is known that an increase in systolic blood pressure (SBP) of 10 mmHg at night increases the risk of death by 21% [15]. Non-dipping profiles were observed more often in PreD only if chronic kidney disease was also present [16].

Hypertensive crisis is defined as a SBP above 180 mmHg and/or diastolic blood pressure (DBP) above 120 mmHg, which includes uncontrolled AH (HU, without TOD—eyes, brain, heart, aorta, kidneys) and hypertensive emergency (with acute TOD) [17–19]. In addition to BP control, rigorous control of all risk factors and screening of damage within the CV system is required. Although total CV risk reduction is the final goal of AH management, treatment according to guidelines, awareness of the seriousness of this problem and the need for a continuous individual and multidisciplinary approach are insufficient and call for change [20].

PreD and non-dipping profiles are significantly underestimated in clinical practice, leaving many patients with high cardiovascular risk and already existing TOD without adequate and timely therapy, especially if they have normal BP values [21,22]. PWV measurement is still relatively inaccessible, and according to current guidelines, its use in daily clinical practice is not recommended [17]. On the other hand, all other mentioned tests are recommended and available in a family medicine setting.

Aim of the Study

The aim of this study is to compare the PWV values in subjects with PreD, non-dipper profiles and arterial hypertension with their values in healthy subjects. We hypothesize that higher FPG values, higher BP levels and a non-dipper profile are associated with higher PWV values and higher CV risk, i.e., TOD.

2. Methods

This cross-sectional study was conducted in four family medicine practices (FMP) of the Health Center Zagreb-West (groups A and B) and at the Emergency department of the Clinical Hospital Merkur (group C) in Zagreb, Croatia from January 2019 to December 2022. We completed an a priori power analysis and the power analysis resulted in 251; however, we recruited 301 Caucasian subjects (153 women and 148 men). Information about a patient's medical history and used medication was collected from the electronic medical record (Medicus.Net system for FMP and Hospital Information System (BIS) in Clinical Hospital Merkur). Subjects were divided into three groups using the 24 h ambulatory blood pressure monitoring (ABPM) findings.

2.1. Groups Depending on Hypertensive Status

- Group A (healthy persons)—subjects were selected by simple random sampling from the list of insured persons in four FMPs without a diagnosis of AH (ICD-10: I10-I15) and with average BP values lower than 130/80 mmHg measured by ABPM.
- Group B (patients with AH without HU)—subjects from four FMPs with a diagnosis of AH (ICD-10: I10-I15) confirmed by ABPM without measured BP values higher than 180 mmHg and/or 120 mmHg in more than five individual measurements and data about HU in the medical history. AH is defined by exceeding the average of all measured BP values above 130 and/or 80 mmHg by APBM and/or taking at least one antihypertensive drug [16,22].
- Group C (patients with HU)—was formed by simple random sampling of patients from the database of patients from Clinical Hospital Merkur who sought emergency medical help due to high BP values. BP values upon arrival at the institution were measured after five minutes of quiet sitting with a one-minute interval between each measurement (three times), and ABPM was set upon discharge. Only those patients whose BP values were measured by a correctly performed ABPM of more than 180 and/or 120 mmHg in more than five individual measurements for 24 h were included.

2.2. Exclusion Criteria

Exclusion criteria included hypertensive emergency, CV event in personal medical history, incomplete data, age below 40 and above 70 years, BMI > 50 kg/m^2, atrial fibrillation, diabetes mellitus, chronic kidney disease G3b, G4 and G5, pregnancy, immunosuppressive, corticosteroid and/or biological therapy, chemotherapy regime in the last five years and expected life expectancy less than six months.

2.3. PWV and ABPM Measurements

A session of 24 h ABPM was performed on a special schedule (from 1 pm to 1 pm the next day, 80 BP measurements) using the BTL Cardiopoint® (BTL, Marlborough, MA, USA) device using an adequate cuff placed on the lower half of the subject's upper arm determined by the circumference of the middle part of the distal half of the upper arm (cuff S = 12 × 22 cm^2 for circumference 22–26 cm, M = 16 × 30 cm^2 for 27–34 cm, L = 16 × 36 cm^2 for 35–44 cm, XL = 16 × 42 cm^2 for 45–52 cm). All subjects were divided into three groups according to the percentage change in night BP value (dipper ≥10%, non-dipper 0–10% and inverse dipper <0%) [23,24]. In case of borderline BP values (e.g., more than five measured SBP values above 170 mmHg, etc.), duration of ABPM shorter than 20 h or less than 70% of correct measurements, ABPM was repeated two weeks after the first measurement [25].

PWV was measured with an Agedio® B900 (IEM, Stolberg, Germany) oscillometric device at a room temperature of 20–25 °C with a suitable cuff in the same previously described manner as in the performance of ABPM. A total of 2 measurements were taken according to specific schedules with subjects (working days between 2 and 6 pm), between which there was a break of 30 s. At the first measurement, brachial SBP and DBP were determined, and at the second, PWV, central SBP (cSBP), central DBP (cDBP), pulse pressure (PP) and AIx. In case of imprecise measurement, the device reports an error, and the procedure was repeated within five minutes of the first measurement.

2.4. Other Procedures

Participants were recruited during their regular provider visits and then scheduled for ABPM, PWV measurements (within ten working days) and a blood draw. A blood draw was performed during the visit (emergency laboratory parameters for group C) or/and the morning after at 7 to 8.30 am (for groups A and B and other parameters for group C). Biochemical parameters in the examinee's serum were determined by sampling 2 tubes of 8–10 mL of venous blood in the emergency hospital laboratory: the first was to determine hematocrit value, the concentration of creatinine, sodium ions, potassium ions and glucose, while the second was for triglycerides, HDL, LDL, total cholesterol and urate (since they could not be performed in an emergency laboratory). For other subjects, the same laboratory parameters were determined through the primary health care laboratory (including lipid status and urate concentration), and the fasting glucose value was repeated after two weeks.

Acute organ damage in the case of HU was ruled out by standard biochemical and radiological examinations of the clinic (X-ray, CT, ultrasound with or without color doppler) and ECG. It includes acute kidney damage, ischemic or hemorrhagic stroke, acute coronary syndrome, acute pulmonary edema, acute left heart failure, hypertensive encephalopathy and aortic dissection. The glomerular filtration rate was assessed using CKD-EPI (Chronic Kidney Disease Epidemiology Collaboration) formula [26].

On the first visit, chronic antihypertensive and hypolipemic therapy was also recorded. Due to the possible effect on the measurements, the medications were not changed until all procedures were completed (if needed). Additionally, all participants were weighed in the office (anthropometric scale Tanita® (TANITA, Stuttgart, Germany)) and had their height and waist circumference measured with a tailor's tape measure. Prediabetes was defined according to the 2017 ADA criteria [1]. Metabolic syndrome was defined by the National Cholesterol Education Program (NCEP) Adult Treatment Panel III (ATP III) criteria updated by the American Heart Association and the National Heart Lung and Blood Institute in 2005 [27].

This study was approved by the Ethics Committee of the Health Center Zagreb-West (Number 251-12-02-21-19) and the Ethics Committee of the Merkur Clinical Hospital (Number 03/1-6063). All participants signed an informed consent to participate in the research.

2.5. Statistical Analysis

The sample size was calculated according to the expected arithmetic means of the PWV values and their standard deviations. Power analysis was performed a priori for ANOVA for special effects and interactions. With significance level $\alpha = 0.05$, effect size (f) = 0.25, and a total of 251 respondents with equally large groups, ANOVA has a test power of $\beta = 95\%$ to recognize differences in two dependent variables between the three observed groups with one predictor [28]. Finally, 301 subjects were recruited.

The normality of the data distribution was checked with the Kolmogorov-Smirnov test. Continuous variables (depending on the distribution) were analyzed with Student's *t*-test, or Mann-Whitney U test, and categorical variables with Pearson's $\chi 2$ test. ANOVA was used in the analysis of dependent variables. In post hoc analysis, we performed Tukey's HSD test to check the differences between the groups. Variables that showed a statistically significant Pearson correlation with PWV were included in the linear regression model. The final linear regression model included PWV as a dependent variable and age, SBP, DBP, heart rate, nocturnal indices, FPG, and GFR as independent variables. A value of $p < 0.05$ is considered statistically significant. The program used for statistical analysis is Statistica v.12.0.

3. Results

In the studied groups, women were significantly older than men (58.11 vs. 54.59 years, $p < 0.001$), had higher PWV (8.74 vs. 8.44 m/s, $p < 0.05$) and AIx values (27.96 vs. 19.35%, $p < 0.001$), but lower SBP (130.85 vs. 136.97 mmHg, $p < 0.01$), DBP (77.26 vs. 84.46 mmHg, $p < 0.001$), triglycerides (1.40 vs. 1.85 mmol/L, $p < 0.01$), uric acid (294.50 vs. 378.52 umol/L, $p < 0.001$) and BMI values (27.24 vs. 28.45 kg/m^2). Differences in FPG (5.68 vs. 5.85 mmol/L in men, $p = 0.268$) and other variables between sexes were not found.

The division of subjects according to the results of ABPM resulted in 77 subjects in group A, 138 in group B and 86 in group C. Group C had a significantly higher number of patients with PreD (74.41%, $p < 0.001$) compared to the other groups (42.75 vs 35.06%, $p = 0.269$) and a significantly higher number of non-dippers (53.48%, $p < 0.001$) compared to other groups (32.61 vs. 29.87%, $p = 0.653$). Other differences are shown in column A in Table 1. There were 21 (15.22%) subjects newly diagnosed with HA in group B, and 23

(26.75%) in group C. A total of 8 (9.30%) subjects in group C were treated with only one antihypertensive drug.

Table 1. —Differences between healthy subjects (group A), patients with regulated arterial hypertension (group B) and patients with untreated hypertension (group C). B—Differences between healthy and prediabetic subjects (right side). All data are listed as number (percentage), mean ± standard deviation or median (interquartile range).

	A					B		
Variable	**All Groups (N = 301)**	**Group A (N = 77)**	**Group B (N = 138)**	**Group C (N = 86)**	***p***	**Healthy (N = 151)**	**Prediabetes (N = 150)**	***p***
Women	153 (50.83%)	49 (63.64%)	67 (48.55%)	37 (43.02%)	0.064 *	85 (56.29%)	68 (45.33%)	0.057 †
Dippers	164 (54.48%)	55 (71.43%)	82 (59.42%)	27 (31.40%)	<0.001 *	87 (57.61%)	77 (51.33%)	0.274 †
Metabolic syndrome	90 (29.90%)	3 (3.89%)	39 (28.26%)	48 (55.81%)	<0.001 *	20 (13.24%)	69 (46.00%)	<0.001 †
Antihypertensive therapy	180 (80.36%) $^{\theta}$	/	117 (84.78%)	63 (73.25%)	0.119 *	85 (56.29%)	98 (65.33%)	0.108 †
Statin therapy	28 (9.31%)	3 (3.89%)	19 (13.77%)	6 (6.98%)	<0.05 *	13 (8.61%)	17 (11.33%)	0.430 †
Current smoking	110 (36.54%)	28 (36.37%)	45 (32.61%)	37 (43.02%)	<0.05 *	46 (30.46%)	64 (42.66%)	<0.05 †
Age (years)	56.37 ± 7.94	54.68 ± 7.65	57.16 ± 7.61	56.72 ± 8.61	0.069 *	55.59 ± 8.56	57.53 ± 7.01	<0.05 ‡
Average SBP (mmHg)	133.89 ±16.72	117.58 ± 7.61	134.02 ± 10.52	149.41 ± 16.52	<0.001 *	130.90 ± 15.62	137.51 ± 17.34	<0.001 ‡
Average DBP (mmHg)	80.82 ± 11.95	71.71 ± 6.73	79.48 ± 8.35	91.80 ± 12.39	<0.001 *	79.36 ± 11.80	82.52 ± 12.07	<0.05 ‡
Average MAP (mmHg)	98.51 ± 12.81	87.00 ± 6.53	97.66 ± 8.37	111.01 ± 12.26	<0.001 *	96.54 ± 12.46	100.85 ± 12.97	<0.01 ‡
Nocturnal indices (%)	10.83 (4.47–15.44)	12.12 (7.08–17.47)	11.16 (5.26–16.38)	6.18 (2.18–12.14)	<0.001 §	10.66 (4.76–15.83)	10.01 (4.17–14.81)	0.358 §
cSBP (mmHg)	129.82 ± 20.87	115.02 ± 11.09	124.34 ± 13.10	153.39 ± 19.06	<0.001 *	124.61 ± 18.29	135.60 ± 22.24	<0.001 ‡
cDBP (mmHg)	90.04 ± 15.54	79.25 ± 9.84	87.50 ± 11.27	104.65 ± 15.41	<0.001 *	87.27 ± 14.62	93.07 ± 16.13	<0.01 ‡
PP (mmHg)	39.94 ± 12.57	36.30 ± 11.68	36.85 ± 8.81	48.81 ± 14.29	<0.001 *	37.24 ± 11.09	42.98 ± 13.42	<0.001 ‡
Heart rate (/min)	73.43 ± 9.24	71.77 ± 7.83	72.41 ± 9.55	76.69 ± 9.28	<0.001 *	73.30 ± 9.91	73.71 ± 8.68	0.444 ‡
GFR (ml/min/1.73 m^2)	89.83 ± 14.52	90.70 ± 13.51	89.59 ± 13.43	89.43 ± 17.01	0.828 *	90.46 ± 13.44	89.19 ± 15.56	0.449 ‡
FPG (mmol/L)	5.76 ± 1.33	5.39 ± 0.61	5.56 ± 0.77	6.41 ± 1.09	<0.001 *	5.04 ± 0.32	6.48 ± 0.56	<0.001 ‡
Potassium (mmol/L)	4.27 ± 0.41	4.37 ± 0.34	4.30 ± 1.18	4.12 ± 0.45	<0.001 *	4.30 ± 0.41	4.23 ± 0.40	0.118 ‡
Total cholesterol (mmol/L)	5.93 ± 1.18	5.94 ± 1.11	5.77 ± 1.18	6.16 ± 1.23	0.062 *	5.78 ± 1.20	6.07 ± 1.15	<0.05 ‡
Non-HDL c (mmol/L)	4.44 ± 1.39	4.23 ± 1.09	4.34 ± 1.13	4.77 ± 1.17	<0.05 *	4.29 ± 1.16	4.58 ± 1.57	<0.01 ‡
Triglycerides (mmol/L)	1.62 ± 0.97	1.1 (0.9–1.6)	1.4 (1.1–1.8)	1.5 (1.1–2.2)	<0.05 §	1.3 (0.9–1.7)	1.5 (1.1–2.1)	<0.01 §
Uric acid (umol/L)	335.99 ± 88.34	295.49 ± 70.16	338.36 ± 84.59	373.39 ± 96.86	<0.001 *	325.36 ± 83.07	348.24 ± 92.93	0.063 ‡
BMI (kg/m^2)	28.15 ± 6.94	24.71 ± 3.42	28.18 ± 4.74	30.34 ± 4.66	<0.001 *	27.24 ± 5.12	28.45 ± 4.51	<0.05 ‡
WC (cm)	94.3 ± 3.3	88.4 ± 2.8	94.2 ± 3.1	101.2 ± 4.6	<0.001 *	94.0 ± 2.4	99.0 ± 3.4	<0.01 ‡
PWV (m/s)	8.59 ± 1.32	7.79 ± 1.10	8.46 ± 1.01	9.60 ± 1.34	<0.001 *	8.26 ± 1.22	8.98 ± 1.31	<0.001 ‡
AIx (%)	22 (15–31)	21 (12–34)	21 (13–31)	24 (21–30)	<0.05 §	22 (13–31)	23 (18–32)	0.247 §

SB*p* = systolic blood pressure; DB*p* = diastolic blood pressure; MA*p* = mean arterial pressure; GFR = glomerular filtration rate; FPG = fasting plasma glucose; PWV = pulse wave velocity; cSB*p* = central systolic blood pressure; cDB*p* = central diastolic blood pressure; P*p* = pulse pressure; AIx = augmentation index; WC = waist circumference; $^{\theta}$ = without group A. * ANOVA; † Pearson χ^2 test; ‡ Student *t*-test; § Mann–Whitney test.

The number of dippers, specifically using nocturnal indices, were comparable between the healthy subjects and those with PreD (Table 1B). In the linear regression model, age, SBP, DBP, nocturnal indices and FPG proved to be independent predictors of PWV values (Table 2).

Table 2. Evaluation of parameters affecting PWV by linear regression analysis. Regression summary for dependent variable PWV: R = 0.839; R^2 = 0.705; Adjusted R^2 = 0.698; F (7.291) = 99.507; $p < 0.001$; Standard Error of estimate: 0.721; N = 301.

	B	Standard Error	T	*p*
Intercept		0.694	−3.495	<0.001
Age	0.736	0.035	20.759	<0.001
SBP	0.222	0.049	4.539	<0.001
DBP	0.109	0.051	2.135	0.034
Nocturnal indices	−0.107	0.459	−3.280	0.001
Heart rate	0.040	0.034	1.189	0.235
GFR	−0.048	0.034	−1.416	0.158
FPG	0.143	0.032	4.433	<0.001

SB*p* = systolic blood pressure; DB*p* = diastolic blood pressure; GFR = glomerular filtration rate; FPG = fasting plasma glucose; PWV = pulse wave velocity.

All dippers had the lowest average PWV values (8.23 m/s), followed by non-dippers with higher average PWV values (8.87 m/s, $p < 0.001$). The highest PWV values were measured in all inverse dippers (9.49 m/s, $p < 0.001$), especially in group C (10.12 m/s). All differences between the examined dipping profiles and hypertension groups are shown in Figure 1.

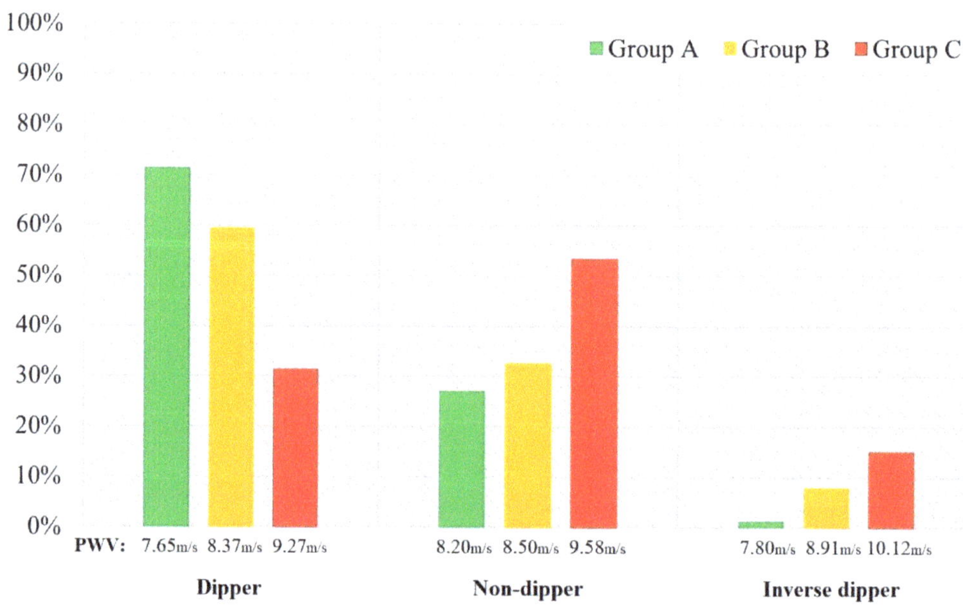

Figure 1. Ratio of subjects with certain dipping profile in examined groups and group pulse wave velocity (PWV) values. Group A = healthy subjects (N = 77); B = subjects with controlled hypertension (N = 138); C = subjects with uncontrolled hypertension (N = 86).

PWV values were statistically much higher in subjects with both PreD and a non-dipper profile compared to subjects without PreD and with normal dipper profile in all three age groups (40–50 years: 8.41 vs. 6.69 m/s, $p < 0.001$; 50–60 years: 8.79 vs. 8.05 m/s, $p < 0.01$; 60–70 years: 10.24 vs. 9.22 m/s, $p < 0.001$). Although statistically insignificant, PWV values were slightly higher in non-dippers without PreD than in dippers with PreD (Figure 2), with no significant gender differences in post hoc analysis and the univariate test of significance (F = 0.80, $p = 0.370$). In PWV analysis among hypertension groups, subjects with PreD and a non-dipper profile had the highest values of all other group subjects without noticeable differences between genders (Table 3).

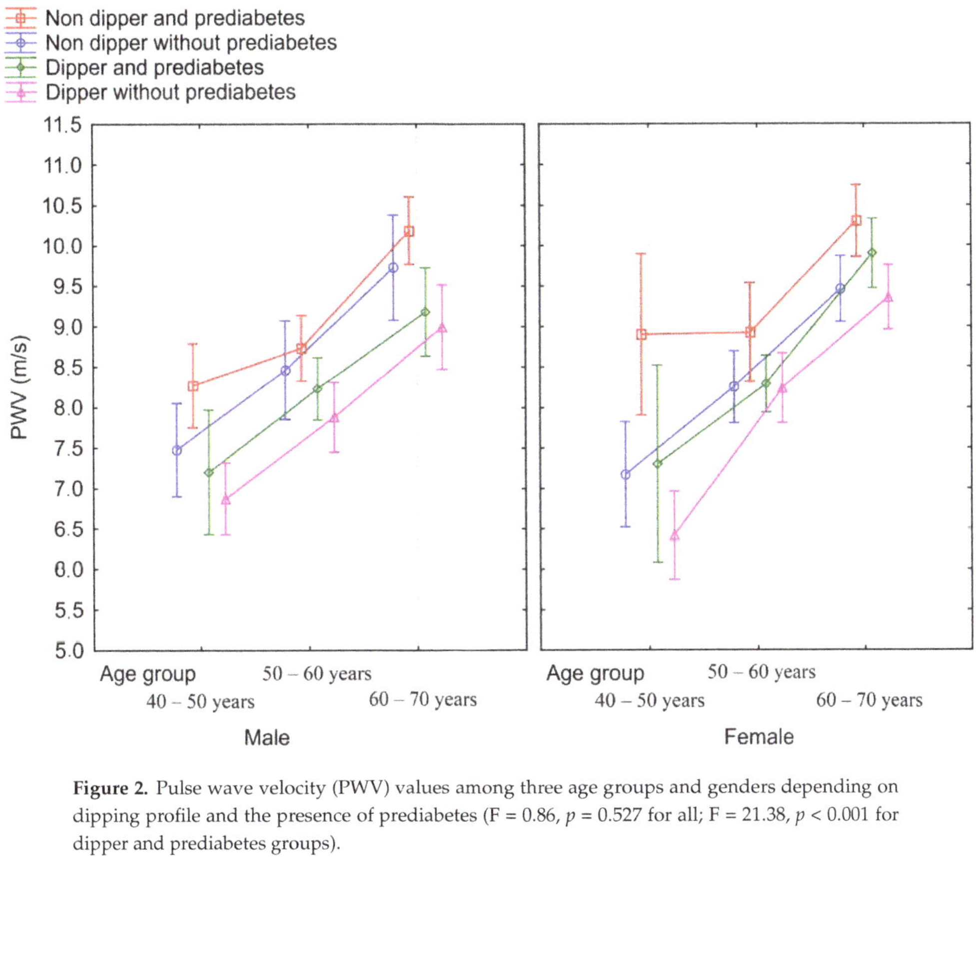

Figure 2. Pulse wave velocity (PWV) values among three age groups and genders depending on dipping profile and the presence of prediabetes (F = 0.86, $p = 0.527$ for all; F = 21.38, $p < 0.001$ for dipper and prediabetes groups).

Table 3. Hypertension groups and PWV values depending on dipping status, prediabetes (PreD) and gender. Values represent means ± standard deviation and were analyzed by one-way ANOVA divided by groups.

	Gender	Non-Dipper and PreD (N = 72)	Dipper and PreD (N = 64)	Non-Dipper without PreD (N = 77)	Dipper without PreD (N = 87)	p
Group A (Healthy subjects)	Male	8.17 ± 1.04	7.90 ± 0.56	7.82 ± 1.14	7.22 ± 0.99	0.904
	Female	9.07 ± 1.04	8.60 ± 0.93	8.34 ± 0.66	7.70 ± 1.30	
Group B (Subjects with controlled hypertension)	Male	8.37 ± 1.16	8.31 ± 1.38	8.22 ± 0.93	7.98 ± 0.92	0.308
	Female	8.90 ± 0.23	8.62 ± 0.90	8.82 ± 0.91	8.32 ± 1.07	
Group C (Subjects with uncontrolled hypertension)	Male	9.42 ± 1.25	9.05 ± 1.50	8.60 ± 0.66	8.12 ± 0.59	0.572
	Female	10.37 ± 1.42	9.90 ± 0.28	10.10 ± 0.79	9.75 ± 1.04	
All groups	Male	9.16 ± 1.42	8.46 ± 1.29	8.35 ± 0.91	7.81 ± 1.01	0.769
	Female	9.71 ± 1.39	8.60 ± 1.16	8.52 ± 1.17	8.31 ± 1.30	

4. Discussion

In this study, PWV was significantly associated with the existence of PreD, nocturnal indices and BP values. PWV values were notably higher in PreD patients, especially in combination with a non-dipper profile in all three age and hypertensive groups. Special attention should be given to the group of apparently healthy subjects (group A) in which as many as 35% of them had PreD and 28% were non-dippers since their PWV values were even higher than in patients with well-controlled AH (group B) in our study. These subjects are often neglected in clinical practice because they seem to have a negligible CV risk, according to SCORE2 charts [29].

If we consider that higher PWV equals higher CV risk (TOD), then patients with PreD and non-dipping profiles in all hypertensive groups had the highest CV risk than all other subjects, which increases with aging [9,30,31]. Knowing that 9 to 50% of persons with PreD will develop T2DM in five years and 70% in ten years, the CV risk will additionally increase, because of which we have to start treating PreD and all CV risk factors immediately [32,33]. Therefore, Yasuno et al. [34] demonstrated high PP and PWV values as predictors of new-onset T2DM in hypertensive patients, independent of the effects of antihypertensive therapy and other risk factors. An American study from 2012 conducted by Mainous et al. [35] and using data from the National Ambulatory Medical Care Survey showed that only 23% of patients diagnosed with PreD were advised to change their lifestyle or were offered metformin. Many years before, the successfulness of lifestyle changes was shown by Tuomilehto et al. [36] who calculated that 22 subjects with PreD must be treated using non-pharmacological interventions in the primary care setting for one year (or five subjects for five years) to prevent one case of diabetes. Furthermore, obesity prevalence in children is growing worldwide and represents another crucial medical problem associated with increased arterial stiffness and BP values leading to accelerated atherosclerosis in early life [8]. Regardless of the age and CV risk, Zheng et al. [14] showed (on 20,355 participants) that avoiding smoking, alcohol non-consumption, low salt intake and increased physical activity (ideal CV health) can reduce PWV and the risk of cardiac and cerebral events.

Besides increased FPG, glycemic variability (GV) is associated with accelerated atherosclerosis even in non-diabetics, independently of conventional risk factors [37]. A study by Tateishi et al. [38] showed a greater GV impact on coronary endothelial dysfunction but no association with peripheral endothelial function. On the other hand, Yu et al. [39] observed CVD development and all-cause death over eight years in non-diabetic patients from a nationwide database of Koreans. They found that the risk of all-cause mortality and early death of CVD was significantly higher in the highest quartile of GV (24% and 21%, respectively). Although Foreman et al. [40] demonstrated the association between higher GV and greater PWV in 853 participants with T2DM, due to the very small number of studies which studied the relationship between GV and PWV, this association requires further investigation. Although our study did not investigate GV, high FPG was associated with significantly higher PWV. GV promotes inflammation and oxidative stress which causes the formation of cross-links of elastin and collagen [41,42]. Finally, the variability of many other CV risk factors (SBP, FPG, total cholesterol and BMI) was found to be an independent predictor of mortality and CV events [43]. Based on all the evidence, addressing all those metabolic risk factors is needed along with lifestyle changes in subjects with high PWV values (high CV risk).

A non-dipping profile is associated with impaired modulation of vascular smooth muscle tone during the night, increased PWV and CV risk [22,44]. The most common comorbidity connected with a non-dipping or inverse dipping profile is obstructive sleep apnea syndrome which should be quickly evaluated and treated [6]. Our results confirm the hypothesis that non-dipping status combined with PreD would lead to even greater PWV values, especially in subjects with uncontrolled arterial hypertension (group C), increasing their CV risk to high or very high [45]. We assume that PreD and non-dipper status did not affect PWV values in group B as expected (as in groups A and C) because of antihypertensive medication's protective effect on the CV system (e.g., ACE inhibitors, ARBs) and good BP regulation [46].

A great problem of everyday clinical practice is the underutilization of CVD prevention. ESH-ESC Guidelines recommend using the SCORE2 model as a minimum requirement. However, TOD is not included in it, making the CV risk stratification imprecise [47]. For example, even 26% of subjects at the time of HU (group C) did not have a diagnosis of AH, while only 7% of subjects in group C were taking statin therapy despite the high CV risk and the guidelines. In our study, patients with uncontrolled AH had the highest PWV values in all age groups, independently of PreD and non-dipper profile, which is why we need to work on better care and treatment of such patients. More precise determination of total CV risk using oscillometric devices for PWV measurement in FMP should be the basis for timely recognition, rational diagnosis and better treatment of AH, reducing GV and FPG, and correcting dipping status and other CV risk factors to reduce the number of CV complications and improve the patient's quality of life.

Strengths and Limitations

The strength of this study is that PWV was also measured in healthy subjects included by strict criteria, always at a similar time of day (2–6 pm) with little differences in air temperature (20–25 °C), which can be extremely important for the accuracy of the measurement [48].

This study has several limitations. For defining PreD, we used average FPG from two measurements. HbA1c and values of albuminuria (an important parameter of TOD) could not be obtained due to practical reasons. In a small number of patients, the ABPM and PWV measurements were not performed on the same day due to the oscillometric device's unavailability. The number of patients with an inverse dipping profile in different groups (especially in the age group 40–50 years) was too small (some were equal to zero) for good analysis using ANOVA. Accordingly, inverse dippers were not included in the ANOVA analysis.

5. Conclusions

Our findings showed significantly higher PWV values in subjects with PreD and non-dipping profile in all three examined hypertension groups, meaning these subjects already have higher CV risk and a greater probability of TOD. This study highlights the relevance of BP evaluation with ABPM in all subjects with PreD and the timely introduction of lifestyle changes and medication when needed. Future studies should assess the impact of lifestyle and medication interventions on PWV values in otherwise healthy subjects with PreD.

Author Contributions: Conceptualization, J.J.; data curation, J.J.; formal analysis, J.J. and Đ.D.; methodology, J.J., V.B.L., T.B. and I.P.; project administration, J.J., Đ.D. and I.P.; resources, T.B. and I.P.; supervision, V.B.L. and I.P.; writing—original draft, J.J. and Đ.D.; writing—review and editing, V.B.L., T.B. and I.P. All authors have read and agreed to the published version of the manuscript.

Funding: This research received no external funding.

Institutional Review Board Statement: This study was approved by the Ethics Committee of the Health Center Zagreb-West and the Ethics Committee of the Merkur Clinical Hospital (Number 03/1-6063). All participants signed an informed consent to participate in the research.

Informed Consent Statement: Informed consent was obtained from all subjects involved in the study.

Data Availability Statement: The data presented in this study are available on request from the corresponding author.

Acknowledgments: We want to thank Ivan Marinović, Ana Vlašić and Nives Bunić for help in collecting the participants for this study, and Marija Zdelar, Mira Bosak and Petra Stipić for assisting in the diagnostic part of the examination.

Conflicts of Interest: The authors declare no conflict of interest.

References

1. American Diabetes Association 2. Classification and Diagnosis of Diabetes. *Diabetes Care* **2017**, *40*, S11–S24. [CrossRef]
2. Authors/Task Force Members; Ryden, L.; Grant, P.J.; Anker, S.D.; Berne, C.; Cosentino, F.; Danchin, N.; Deaton, C.; Escaned, J.; Hammes, H.P.; et al. ESC Guidelines on Diabetes, Pre-Diabetes, and Cardiovascular Diseases Developed in Collaboration with the EASD. The Task Force on Diabetes, Pre-Diabetes, and Cardiovascular Diseases of the European Society of Cardiology (ESC) and Developed in Collaboration with the European Association for the Study of Diabetes (EASD). *Rev. Esp. Cardiol. Engl. Ed.* **2014**, *67*, 136. [CrossRef]
3. Færch, K.; Vistisen, D.; Johansen, N.B.; Jørgensen, M.E. Cardiovascular Risk Stratification and Management in Pre-Diabetes. *Curr. Diabetes Rep.* **2014**, *14*, 493. [CrossRef] [PubMed]
4. Ford, E.S.; Zhao, G.; Li, C. Pre-Diabetes and the Risk for Cardiovascular Disease. *J. Am. Coll. Cardiol.* **2010**, *55*, 1310–1317. [CrossRef] [PubMed]
5. Gupta, A.K.; Greenway, F.L.; Cornelissen, G.; Pan, W.; Halberg, F. Prediabetes Is Associated with Abnormal Circadian Blood Pressure Variability. *J. Hum. Hypertens.* **2008**, *22*, 627–633. [CrossRef] [PubMed]
6. Roth, G.A.; Mensah, G.A.; Johnson, C.O.; Addolorato, G.; Ammirati, E.; Baddour, L.M.; Barengo, N.C.; Beaton, A.Z.; Benjamin, E.J.; Benziger, C.P.; et al. Global Burden of Cardiovascular Diseases and Risk Factors, 1990–2019. *J. Am. Coll. Cardiol.* **2020**, *76*, 2982–3021. [CrossRef]
7. de Rezende Mikael , L.; de Paiva, A.M.G.; Gomes, M.M.; Sousa, A.L.L.; Jardim, P.C.B.V.; de Oliveira Vitorino, P.V.; Euzébio, M.B.; de Sousa, W.M.; Barroso, W.K.S. Vascular Aging and Arterial Stiffness. *Arq. Bras. Cardiol.* **2017**, *109*, 253–258. [CrossRef]
8. Mihuta, M.S.; Paul, C.; Borlea, A.; Cepeha, C.M.; Velea, I.P.; Mozos, I.; Stoian, D. The Oscillometric Pulse Wave Analysis Is Useful in Evaluating the Arterial Stiffness of Obese Children with Relevant Cardiometabolic Risks. *J. Clin. Med.* **2022**, *11*, 5078. [CrossRef]
9. Vlachopoulos, C.; Aznaouridis, K.; Stefanadis, C. Prediction of Cardiovascular Events and All-Cause Mortality with Arterial Stiffness. *J. Am. Coll. Cardiol.* **2010**, *55*, 1318–1327. [CrossRef]
10. Vasan, R.S.; Short, M.I.; Niiranen, T.J.; Xanthakis, V.; DeCarli, C.; Cheng, S.; Seshadri, S.; Mitchell, G.F. Interrelations between Arterial Stiffness, Target Organ Damage, and Cardiovascular Disease Outcomes. *J. Am. Heart Assoc.* **2019**, *8*, e012141. [CrossRef]
11. Aristizábal-Ocampo, D.; Espíndola-Fernández, D.; Gallo-Villegas, J. Pulse Wave Velocity Reference Values in 3,160 Adults Referred to a Hypertension Clinic for 24-Hour Ambulatory Blood Pressure Monitoring. *Clin. Exp. Hypertens.* **2019**, *41*, 759–765. [CrossRef] [PubMed]
12. Loehr, L.R.; Meyer, M.L.; Poon, A.K.; Selvin, E.; Palta, P.; Tanaka, H.; Pankow, J.S.; Wright, J.D.; Griswold, M.E.; Wagenknecht, L.E.; et al. Prediabetes and Diabetes Are Associated with Arterial Stiffness in Older Adults: The ARIC Study. *Am. J. Hypertens.* **2016**, *29*, 1038–1045. [CrossRef]
13. Horton, W.B.; Jahn, L.A.; Hartline, L.M.; Aylor, K.W.; Patrie, J.T.; Barrett, E.J. Insulin Increases Central Aortic Stiffness in Response to Hyperglycemia in Healthy Humans: A Randomized Four-Arm Study. *Diabetes Vasc. Dis. Res.* **2021**, *18*, 147916412110110. [CrossRef]
14. Zheng, X.; Zhang, R.; Liu, X.; Zhao, H.; Liu, H.; Gao, J.; Wu, Y.; Wu, S. Association between Cumulative Exposure to Ideal Cardiovascular Health and Arterial Stiffness. *Atherosclerosis* **2017**, *260*, 56–62. [CrossRef] [PubMed]
15. Dolan, E.; Stanton, A.A.N.; Thijs, L.M.S. Superiority of Ambulatory over Clinic Blood Pressure Measurement in Predicting Mortality: The Dublin Outcome Study. *Hypertension* **2005**, *46*, 156–161. [CrossRef] [PubMed]
16. Obayashi, K.; Saeki, K.; Kurumatani, N. Nighttime BP in Elderly Individuals with Prediabetes/Diabetes with and without CKD: The HEIJO-KYO Study. *Clin. J. Am. Soc. Nephrol.* **2016**, *11*, 867–874. [CrossRef]
17. Mancia, G.; Rosei, E.A.; Azizi, M.; Burnier, M.; Clement, D.L.; Coca, A.; de Simone, G.; Dominiczak, A.; Kahan, T.; Mahfoud, F.; et al. 2018 ESC/ESH Guidelines for the Management of Arterial Hypertension. *Eur. Heart J.* **2018**, *39*, 3021–3104.
18. Patel, K.K.; Young, L.; Howell, E.H.; Hu, B.; Rutecki, G.; Thomas, G.; Rothberg, M.B. Characteristics and Outcomes of Patients Presenting with Hypertensive Urgency in the Office Setting. *JAMA Intern. Med.* **2016**, *176*, 981. [CrossRef]

19. Astarita, A.; Covella, M.; Vallelonga, F.; Cesareo, M.; Totaro, S.; Ventre, L.; Aprà, F.; Veglio, F.; Milan, A. Hypertensive Emergencies and Urgencies in Emergency Departments: A Systematic Review and Meta-Analysis. *J. Hypertens.* **2020**, *38*, 1203–1210. [CrossRef]
20. Levy, P.D.; Mahn, J.J.; Miller, J.; Shelby, A.; Brody, A.; Davidson, R.; Burla, M.J.; Marinica, A.; Carroll, J.; Purakal, J.; et al. Blood Pressure Treatment and Outcomes in Hypertensive Patients without Acute Target Organ Damage: A Retrospective Cohort. *Am. J. Emerg. Med.* **2015**, *33*, 1219–1224. [CrossRef]
21. Zand, A.; Ibrahim, K.; Patham, B. Prediabetes: Why Should We Care? *Methodist DeBakey Cardiovasc. J.* **2018**, *14*, 289–297. [CrossRef] [PubMed]
22. Cicek, Y.; Durakoglugil, M.E.; Kocaman, S.A.; Cetin, M.; Erdogan, T.; Dogan, S.; Ugurlu, Y.; Canga, A. Non-Dipping Pattern in Untreated Hypertensive Patients Is Related to Increased Pulse Wave Velocity Independent of Raised Nocturnal Blood Pressure. *Blood Press.* **2013**, *22*, 34–38. [CrossRef] [PubMed]
23. O'Brien, E.; Parati, G.; Stergiou, G.; Asmar, R.; Beilin, L.; Bilo, G.; Clement, D.; de la Sierra, A.; de Leeuw, P.; Dolan, E.; et al. European Society of Hypertension Position Paper on Ambulatory Blood Pressure Monitoring. *J. Hypertens.* **2013**, *31*, 1731–1768. [CrossRef] [PubMed]
24. Fagard, R.H. Dipping Pattern of Nocturnal Blood Pressure in Patients with Hypertension. *Expert Rev. Cardiovasc. Ther.* **2009**, *7*, 599–605. [CrossRef] [PubMed]
25. Gaborieau, V.; Delarche, N.; Gosse, P. Ambulatory Blood Pressure Monitoring versus Self-Measurement of Blood Pressure at Home: Correlation with Target Organ Damage. *J. Hypertens.* **2008**, *26*, 1919–1927. [CrossRef]
26. Levey, A.S.; Stevens, L.A.; Schmid, C.H.; Iii, A.F.C.; Feldman, H.I.; Kusek, J.W.; Eggers, P.; Coresh, J. A New Equation to Estimate Glomerular Filtration Rate. *Ann. Intern. Med.* **2009**, *150*, 604–612. [CrossRef]
27. Howard, W.J. Diagnosis and Management of the Metabolic Syndrome: An American Heart Association/National Heart, Lung, and Blood Institute Scientific Statement. *Yearb. Endocrinol.* **2006**, *2006*, 113–114. [CrossRef]
28. Cohen, J. *Statistical Power Analysis for the Behavioral Sciences*, 2nd ed.; L. Erlbaum Associates: Hillsdale, NJ, USA, 1988, ISBN 978-0-8058-0283-2.
29. SCORE2 Working Group and ESC Cardiovascular Risk Collaboration. SCORE2 Risk Prediction Algorithms: New Models to Estimate 10-Year Risk of Cardiovascular Disease in Europe. *Eur. Heart J.* **2021**, *42*, 2439–2454. [CrossRef]
30. Gagliardino, J.J.; Salazar, M.R.; Espeche, W.G.; Tolosa Chapasian, P.E.; Gomez Garizoain, D.; Olano, R.D.; Stavile, R.N.; Balbín, E.; Martinez, C.; Leiva Sisnieguez, B.C.; et al. Arterial Stiffness: Its Relation with Prediabetes and Metabolic Syndrome and Possible Pathogenesis. *J. Clin. Med.* **2021**, *10*, 3251. [CrossRef]
31. Kim, J.M.; Kim, S.S.; Kim, I.J.; Kim, J.H.; Kim, B.H.; Kim, M.K.; Lee, S.H.; Lee, C.W.; Kim, M.C.; Ahn, J.H.; et al. Arterial Stiffness Is an Independent Predictor for Risk of Mortality in Patients with Type 2 Diabetes Mellitus: The REBOUND Study. *Cardiovasc. Diabetol.* **2020**, *19*, 143. [CrossRef]
32. Bertram, M.Y.; Vos, T. Quantifying the Duration of Pre-Diabetes. *Aust. N. Z. J. Public Health* **2010**, *34*, 311–314. [CrossRef] [PubMed]
33. Zhang, X.; Gregg, E.W.; Williamson, D.F.; Barker, L.E.; Thomas, W.; Bullard, K.M., Imperatore, G.; Williams, D.E.; Albright, A.L. A1C Level and Future Risk of Diabetes: A Systematic Review. *Diabetes Care* **2010**, *33*, 1665–1673. [CrossRef]
34. Yasuno, S.; Ueshima, K.; Oba, K.; Fujimoto, A.; Hirata, M.; Ogihara, T.; Saruta, T.; Nakao, K. Is Pulse Pressure a Predictor of New-Onset Diabetes in High-Risk Hypertensive Patients? *Diabetes Care* **2010**, *33*, 1122–1127. [CrossRef] [PubMed]
35. Mainous, A.G.; Tanner, R.J.; Baker, R. Prediabetes Diagnosis and Treatment in Primary Care. *J. Am. Board Fam. Med.* **2016**, *29*, 283–285. [CrossRef] [PubMed]
36. Tuomilehto, J.; Lindström, J.; Eriksson, J.G.; Valle, T.T.; Hämäläinen, H.; Ilanne-Parikka, P.; Keinänen-Kiukaanniemi, S.; Laakso, M.; Louheranta, A.; Rastas, M.; et al. Prevention of Type 2 Diabetes Mellitus by Changes in Lifestyle among Subjects with Impaired Glucose Tolerance. *N. Engl. J. Med.* **2001**, *344*, 1343–1350. [CrossRef]
37. Nusca, A.; Tuccinardi, D.; Albano, M.; Cavallaro, C.; Ricottini, E.; Manfrini, S.; Pozzilli, P.; Di Sciascio, G. Glycemic Variability in the Development of Cardiovascular Complications in Diabetes. *Diabetes Metab. Res. Rev.* **2018**, *34*, e3047. [CrossRef]
38. Tateishi, K.; Saito, Y.; Kitahara, H.; Kobayashi, Y. Impact of Glycemic Variability on Coronary and Peripheral Endothelial Dysfunction in Patients with Coronary Artery Disease. *J. Cardiol.* **2022**, *79*, 65–70. [CrossRef]
39. Yu, J.H.; Han, K.; Park, S.; Lee, D.Y.; Nam, G.E.; Seo, J.A.; Kim, S.G.; Baik, S.H.; Park, Y.G.; Kim, S.M.; et al. Effects of Long-Term Glycemic Variability on Incident Cardiovascular Disease and Mortality in Subjects without Diabetes: A Nationwide Population-Based Study. *Medicine* **2019**, *98*, e16317. [CrossRef]
40. Foreman, Y.D.; van Doorn, W.P.T.M.; Schaper, N.C.; van Greevenbroek, M.M.J.; van der Kallen, C.J.H.; Henry, R.M.A.; Koster, A.; Eussen, S.J.P.M.; Wesselius, A.; Reesink, K.D.; et al. Greater Daily Glucose Variability and Lower Time in Range Assessed with Continuous Glucose Monitoring Are Associated with Greater Aortic Stiffness: The Maastricht Study. *Diabetologia* **2021**, *64*, 1880–1892. [CrossRef]
41. Ceriello, A.; Kilpatrick, E.S. Glycemic Variability: Both Sides of the Story. *Diabetes Care* **2013**, *36*, S272–S275. [CrossRef]
42. Prenner, S.B.; Chirinos, J.A. Arterial Stiffness in Diabetes Mellitus. *Atherosclerosis* **2015**, *238*, 370–379. [CrossRef]
43. Kim, M.K.; Han, K.; Park, Y.-M.; Kwon, H.-S.; Kang, G.; Yoon, K.-H.; Lee, S.-H. Associations of Variability in Blood Pressure, Glucose and Cholesterol Concentrations, and Body Mass Index with Mortality and Cardiovascular Outcomes in the General Population. *Circulation* **2018**, *138*, 2627–2637. [CrossRef]

44. Jerrard-Dunne, P.; Mahmud, A.; Feely, J. Circadian Blood Pressure Variation: Relationship between Dipper Status and Measures of Arterial Stiffness. *J. Hypertens.* **2007**, *25*, 1233–1239. [CrossRef]
45. Ben-Shlomo, Y.; Spears, M.; Boustred, C.; May, M.; Anderson, S.G.; Benjamin, E.J.; Boutouyrie, P.; Cameron, J.; Chen, C.-H.; Cruickshank, J.K.; et al. Aortic Pulse Wave Velocity Improves Cardiovascular Event Prediction. *J. Am. Coll. Cardiol.* **2014**, *63*, 636–646. [CrossRef]
46. Li, X.; Chang, P.; Wang, Q.; Hu, H.; Bai, F.; Li, N.; Yu, J. Effects of Angiotensin-Converting Enzyme Inhibitors on Arterial Stiffness: A Systematic Review and Meta-Analysis of Randomized Controlled Trials. *Cardiovasc. Ther.* **2020**, *2020*, 7056184. [CrossRef]
47. Redon, J. Global Cardiovascular Risk Assessment: Strengths and Limitations. *High Blood Press. Cardiovasc. Prev.* **2016**, *23*, 87–90. [CrossRef]
48. Podrug, M.; Šunjić, B.; Bekavac, A.; Koren, P.; Đogaš, V.; Mudnić, I.; Boban, M.; Jerončić, A. The Effects of Experimental, Meteorological, and Physiological Factors on Short-Term Repeated Pulse Wave Velocity Measurements, and Measurement Difficulties: A Randomized Crossover Study with Two Devices. *Front. Cardiovasc. Med.* **2023**, *9*, 993971. [CrossRef]

biomedicines

MDPI

Article

The Impact of BMI Changes on the Incidence of Glomerular Hematuria in Korean Adults: A Retrospective Study Based on the NHIS-HEALS Cohort

Yu-Jin Kwon [1], Mina Kim [2], Hasung Kim [2] and Jung Eun Lee [3,*]

1 Department of Family Medicine, Yongin Severance Hospital, Yonsei University College of Medicine, Seoul 03722, Republic of Korea; digda3@yuhs.ac
2 Data Science Team, Hanmi Pharm. Co., Ltd., Seoul 05545, Republic of Korea; mina.kim92@hanmi.co.kr (M.K.); hasung@hanmi.co.kr (H.K.)
3 Division of Nephrology, Department of Internal Medicine, Yongin Severance Hospital, Yonsei University College of Medicine, Seoul 03722, Republic of Korea
* Correspondence: sw0615@yuhs.ac

Abstract: Obesity and recurrent hematuria are known risk factors for chronic kidney disease. However, there has been controversy on the association between obesity and glomerular hematuria. This study aimed to investigate the association between body mass index (BMI) and weight change and recurrent and persistent hematuria in glomerular disease using a large-scale, population-based Korean cohort. Data were collected from the National Health Insurance Service-National Health Screening Cohort. Cox proportional hazards regression analysis was used to calculate hazard ratios (HRs) and 95% confidence intervals (CIs) for recurrent and persistent hematuria in glomerular disease according to the BMI group. Compared with the BMI 23–25 kg/m^2 group, the HR (95% CI) for incident recurrent and persistent hematuria in glomerular disease was 0.921 (0.831–1.021) in the BMI <23 kg/m^2 group, 0.915 (0.823–1.018) in the BMI 25–30 kg/m^2 group, and 1.151 (0.907–1.462) in the BMI ≥30 kg/m^2 group. Compared with the stable weight group, the HRs (95% CIs) for incident recurrent and persistent hematuria in glomerular disease were 1.364 (1.029–1.808) and 0.985 (0.733–1.325) in the significant weight loss and gain groups, respectively. Despite adjusting for confounders, this result remained significant. Baseline BMI was not associated with the risk of incident recurrent and persistent hematuria in glomerular disease. Weight loss greater than 10% was associated with the incidence of recurrent and persistent hematuria in glomerular disease. Therefore, maintaining an individual's weight could help prevent recurrent and persistent hematuria in glomerular disease in middle-aged and older Korean adults.

Keywords: body mass index; weight loss; hematuria; glomerular disease; kidney disease

1. Introduction

Hematuria is the presence of red blood cells (RBCs) in the urine. These RBCs originate from the glomeruli, renal tubules, interstitium, and urinary tract [1]. The presence of glomerular hematuria is a marker of glomerular filtration barrier dysfunction or damage and results in RBCs with irregular shapes in the urine [2,3]. The prevalence of glomerular hematuria in the general population ranges from 0.18% to 38.7% [3]. A Korean study using data from Korea's national health nutrition examination survey reported that 31.8% of participants aged 10 years and older had isolated hematuria [4]. Recent research suggested that glomerular hematuria promotes oxidative stress, inflammation, and kidney injury [3]. Vivante et al. reported that persistent microscopic hematuria in young adults was significantly associated with the incidence of end-stage renal disease (ESRD) over a 22-year follow-up period [5].

IgA nephropathy (IgAN) is the most common primary glomerular disease worldwide and accounts for half of the glomerular diseases diagnosed by renal biopsy conducted after microscopic hematuria is detected via urinary screening programs [6,7]. Although hematuria is not a specific characteristic of IgAN, recurrent and persistent hematuria is one of the typical symptoms.

Several studies have reported that a high body mass index (BMI) induces enlargement and ultrastructural modification of glomeruli [8]. Obesity leads to the development of kidney disease via direct and indirect mechanisms [9]. Adiposity affects the kidney directly by altering adipokines, such as leptin, resistin, and adiponectin, increasing inflammatory cytokines; oxidative stress; insulin resistance; and activating the renin-angiotensin-aldosterone system [10]. Increased renal metabolic demands with increased body weight result in glomerular hyperfiltration, hypertrophy, and focal or segmental glomerulosclerosis [11]. Obesity also indirectly affects kidneys through the development of metabolic syndrome, diabetes, hypertension, and dyslipidemia [12]. Previous studies suggested that reducing body weight could improve the outcomes of kidney diseases [13,14]. A single-center cohort study [15] reported that low BMI is a significant risk factor for kidney disease progression in IgAN. Another study showed that weight loss is associated with worse outcomes in patients with chronic kidney diseases (CKD) [16]. However, some studies did not find any association between BMI and IgAN progression [17–19]. Currently, the literature shows inconsistent results on associations between BMI and IgAN progression. Furthermore, the role of body weight changes in the incidence of IgAN or glomerular disease with hematuria is still unclear.

Thus, this study aimed to investigate the association between baseline BMI and BMI changes and the incidence of recurrent and persistent hematuria in glomerular disease.

2. Materials and Methods

2.1. Data Source

Data were collected from the Korean National Health Insurance Service-National Health Screening Cohort (NHIS-HEALS) from 2002 to 2015 [20]. Detailed information about the NHIS-HEALS was previously published [20]. The NHIS-HEALS is the national health screening program of Korea, which is designed to prevent and detect non-communicable diseases and health risk factors. The screening program was conducted at least every 2 years among participants aged between 40 and 79 years from 2002 and followed up through 31 December 2015. The Institutional Review Board (IRB) of Yongin Severance Hospital approved the present study (IRB No: 9-2020-0009), which was conducted according to the guidelines of the Declaration of Helsinki.

2.2. Study Population

To diminish any potential effects, participants who underwent health screening in 2002 were excluded. The results on the presence of hematuria by urine dipstick were collected until 31 December 2008. In total, 486,055 participants who underwent their first health screening from 1 January 2003 to 31 December 2008 were included in this study. The follow-up period was from 1 January 2003 to 31 December 2015. Individuals who (1) had proteinuria/hematuria, trace or above, by urine dipstick (n = 59,902); (2) were diagnosed with recurrent and persistent hematuria in glomerular disease (10th edition of the International Classification of Diseases [ICD-10] codes N02.0–N02.8) (n = 231); (3) were diagnosed with malignant neoplasia (ICD-10 codes C), CKD, or ESRD (ICD codes N180, N181, N182, N183, N184, N185, N189) (n = 16,318); and (4) had missing data for age, sex, BMI, or other variables (n = 23,162) at the time of enrollment were excluded. Finally, 386,422 participants were included. The data management is described in Figure 1.

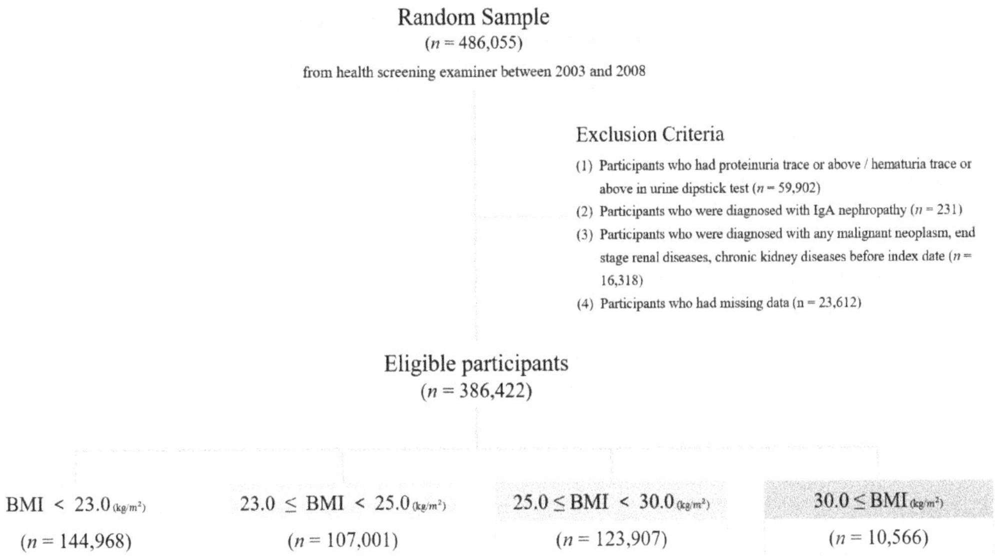

Figure 1. Flow chart of study population.

2.3. *Definition of Recurrent and Persistent Hematuria*

The outcome of this study was recurrent and persistent hematuria in glomerular disease. Data of participants who were diagnosed with recurrent and persistent hematuria as those who were newly diagnosed with ICD codes N02.0–N02.8 from 1 January 2003 to 31 December 2015 were analyzed. These codes are representative codes for IgAN in Korea. The details of the ICD-codes are as follows: N02.0, recurrent and persistent hematuria with minor glomerular abnormality, N02.1, recurrent and persistent hematuria with focal and segmental glomerular lesions; N02.2, recurrent and persistent hematuria with diffuse membranous glomerulonephritis; N02.3, recurrent and persistent hematuria with diffuse mesangial proliferative glomerulonephritis; N02.4, recurrent and persistent hematuria with diffuse endocapillary proliferative glomerulonephritis; N02.5, recurrent and persistent hematuria with diffuse mesangiocapillary glomerulonephritis; N02.6, recurrent and persistent hematuria with dense deposit disease; N02.7, recurrent and persistent hematuria with diffuse crescentic glomerulonephritis; and N02.8, recurrent and persistent hematuria with other morphologic changes.

2.4. *Classification of BMI at Baseline and Definition of BMI Changes*

BMI was calculated as body weight divided by height squared (kg/m^2). Baseline BMI was defined as BMI measured at the first health examination from 2003 to 2008. Baseline BMI was categorized into four groups according to the 2018 Korean Society for the Study of Obesity Guidelines: <23 kg/m^2, 23 to <25 kg/m^2, 25 to <30 kg/m^2, and ≥30 kg/m^2 [21]. Reference BMI was set at 23–25 kg/m^2.

The mean follow-up duration was 6 years. Follow-up BMI was defined as the last checked BMI within 6 years. The BMI change was calculated as the nearest BMI at the end of the follow-up minus the baseline BMI. Patients who had missing follow-up data for BMI within 6 years and those who were diagnosed with recurrent and persistent hematuria in glomerular disease within 6 years were excluded. The flow chart is presented in Supplementary Figure S1. In this analysis, only the incidence of recurrent and persistent hematuria in glomerular disease that occurred after 6 years was considered. The BMI changes during the follow-up period were defined as follows: (follow-up BMI-baseline

BMI) $\times$ 100/baseline BMI. The BMI changes were categorized into quartiles: $<-3.33\%$ (Q1), -3.33–0% (Q2), 0–3.59% (Q3), and $\geq$3.59% (Q4).

Moreover, BMI changes were classified into three groups: weight loss ($<-10\%$), stable weight (-10% to < 10%), and weight gain ($\geq$10%) groups. The reference groups were set as 0–3.59% (Q3) or -10% to <10%.

2.5. Variables

The variables included in the analysis were age, sex, blood pressure (BP), blood glucose level, total cholesterol level, smoking status, alcohol consumption, physical activity, hypertension, diabetes, dyslipidemia, and income status. For these variables, the values measured at the first screening were considered. For the smoking status, the participants were categorized as non-smokers, ex-smokers, or current smokers. Alcohol consumption was categorized into three groups: "rare", less than twice per month; "sometimes", twice per month to twice per week; and "often", more than twice per week. Physical activity level was categorized into three groups: 'rare', did not exercise; 'sometimes', exercised 1–4 times per week; and "regular", exercised more than five times per week. Economic status was categorized into three groups based on individual income percentile: "low", 0–30th percentile; "middle", 40–70th percentile; and "high", 80–100th percentile. Hypertension was defined as ICD I10, I11, I12, I13, I15; diabetes, ICD E10–14; and dyslipidemia, ICD E78.

2.6. Statistical Analysis

All data are presented as the number of participants (%) or the mean $\pm$ standard deviation as appropriate for each variable. To compare the baseline characteristics across the BMI groups, a one-way analysis of variance was used for continuous variables, and the chi-squared test was used for categorical variables. A Cox proportional hazard spline plot was used to assess associations between baseline BMI and BMI changes and the incidence of recurrent and persistent hematuria. The incidence per 1000 person-years was calculated for each group. Cox proportional hazards regression models were used to determine the hazard ratio (HR) and 95% confidence interval (CI) for the incidence of recurrent and persistent hematuria in glomerular disease. An age and sex-adjusted model was set. All multivariable models were adjusted for smoking, alcohol drinking, physical activity, hypertension, diabetes, and dyslipidemia. All p-values were two-sided, and p-values < 0.05 were considered statistically significant. All statistical analyses were performed using SAS version 9.4 (SAS Institute Inc., Cary, NC, USA) and R version 3.5.2 (The R Foundation for Statistical Computing, Vienna, Austria; http://www.R-project.org/ (accessed on 28 February 2022)).

3. Results

Table 1 shows the demographic characteristics of the study cohort stratified by BMI category. Those with higher BMI were older, more likely to be women, and had a higher mean systolic BP, diastolic BP, fasting blood glucose, and total cholesterol. Those with lower BMI were more likely to be current smokers, consume more alcohol, and have a higher household income status.

During the mean follow-up of 6 years, there were 2254 incidents of recurrent and persistent hematuria in glomerular disease events. The incidence in the BMI < 23 kg/m^2 group was 0.50/1000 person-years; BMI 23–25 kg/m^2, 0.54/1000 person-years; BMI 25–30 kg/m^2, 0.50/1000 person-years; and BMI $\geq$ 30 kg/m^2, 0.63/1000 person-years. A multivariable Cox proportional hazards regression model was conducted to determine the relationship between BMI and the incidence of recurrent and persistent hematuria in glomerular disease (Table 2).

Table 1. Baseline characteristics of the study population according to baseline BMI criteria.

	Baseline Body Mass Index				
	<23.0 kg/m²	**23.0–25.0 kg/m²**	**25.0–30.0 kg/m²**	**≥30.0 kg/m²**	*p*
N	144,968	107,001	123,907	10,566	<0.001
Male, *n* (%)	78,341 (54.0)	62,566 (58.5)	72,201 (58.3)	4403 (41.7)	<0.001
Age, years	53.8 ± 10.0	53.5 ± 9.2	53.8 ± 9.0	54.3 ± 9.1	<0.001
BMI, kg/m²	21.1 ± 1.4	24.0 ± 0.6	26.7 ± 1.3	31.8 ± 2.7	<0.001
SBP, mmHg	123.2 ± 17.5	123.4 ± 17.4	130.6 ± 17.4	135.5 ± 18.0	<0.001
DBP, mmHg	77.0 ± 11.2	77.1 ± 11.2	81.7 ± 11.3	84.3 ± 11.7	<0.001
Glucose, mg/dL	95.2 ± 30.3	95.6 ± 30.1	100.5 ± 32.0	104.8 ± 34.9	<0.001
Cholesterol, mg/dL	193.2 ± 36.3	193.8 ± 36.3	205.6 ± 37.8	209.9 ± 38.0	<0.001
Smoking status, *n* (%)					<0.001
Non-smoker	96,973 (66.9)	71,537 (66.9)	83,662 (67.5)	8044 (76.1)	
Ex-smoker	11,056 (7.6)	10,527 (9.8)	12,800 (10.3)	780 (7.4)	
Current smoker	37,539 (25.9)	24,937 (23.3)	27,445 (22.1)	1742 (16.5)	
Alcohol drinking, *n* (%)					<0.001
Rare	84,398 (58.2)	58,848 (55.0)	67,889 (54.8)	6718 (63.6)	
Sometimes	43,726 (30.2)	35,885 (33.5)	41,466 (33.5)	2905 (27.5)	
Often	16,844 (11.6)	12,268 (11.5)	14,552 (11.7)	943 (8.9)	
Physical activity, *n* (%)					<0.001
Rare	83,805 (57.8)	55,438 (51.8)	64,800 (52.3)	6245 (59.1)	
Sometimes	47,864 (33.0)	40,175 (37.5)	45,723 (36.9)	3255 (30.8)	
Regular	13,299 (9.2)	11,388 (10.6)	13,381 (10.8)	1066 (10.1)	
Income status, *n* (%)					<0.001
Low	33,995 (23.5)	22,981 (21.5)	26,689 (21.5)	2669 (25.3)	
Middle	47,684 (32.9)	33,438 (31.3)	40,086 (32.4)	3759 (35.6)	
High	63,289 (43.7)	50,582 (47.3)	57,132 (46.1)	4138 (39.2)	
Comorbidities, *n* (%)					<0.001
Hypertension	22,629 (15.6)	23,270 (21.7)	35,900 (29.0)	4455 (42.2)	
Diabetes	15,649 (10.8)	14,349 (13.4)	19,586 (15.8)	2301 (21.8)	
Dyslipidemia	14,844 (10.2)	14,805 (13.8)	21,260 (17.2)	2307 (21.8)	

BMI, body mass index; SBP, systolic BP; DBP, diastolic BP.

Table 2. Hazard ratios (HRs) and 95% confidence intervals (CIs) for the incidence of recurrent and persistent hematuria in glomerular disease according to body mass index (BMI) status.

	Baseline BMI			
	<23.0 kg/m²	**23.0–25.0 kg/m²**	**25.0–30.0 kg/m²**	**≥30.0 kg/m²**
Total No.	144,968	107,001	123,907	10,566
Event	814	662	703	75
Person-years	1,626,690.04	1,217,843.1	1,412,926.53	119,835.45
IR (per 1000)	0.50	0.54	0.50	0.63
Crude HR	0.921 (0.831–1.021)	1.00 (reference)	0.915 (0.823–1.018)	1.151 (0.907–1.462)
Age- and sex-adjusted HR	0.913 (0.824–1.012)	1.00 (reference)	0.907 (0.816–1.009)	1.10 (0.867–1.398)
Fully adjusted HR	0.946 (0.853–1.049)	1.00 (reference)	0.885 (0.795–0.985)	1.033 (0.812–1.315)

BMI, body mass index; IR, incident rate; HR, hazard ratio; 95% CI, 95% confidence interval. Fully adjusted model: adjusted for age, sex, smoking, alcohol drinking, physical activity, hypertension, diabetes, and dyslipidemia.

Compared to the BMI 23–25 kg/m² group, the HR (95% CI) for incident recurrent and persistent hematuria in glomerular disease was 0.921 (0.831–1.021) in the BMI < 23 kg/m² group; BMI 25–30 kg/m² group, 0.915 (0.823–1.018); and BMI ≥ 30 kg/m², 1.151 (0.907–1.462). The model was adjusted for age and sex; however, there were no significant associations between BMI and the incidence of recurrent and persistent hematuria. Furthermore, after adjusting for age, sex, smoking, alcohol drinking, physical activity, hypertension, diabetes, and dyslipidemia, the results remained insignificant. Figure 2A shows a spline curve for incident recurrent and persistent hematuria in glomerular disease according to baseline BMI.

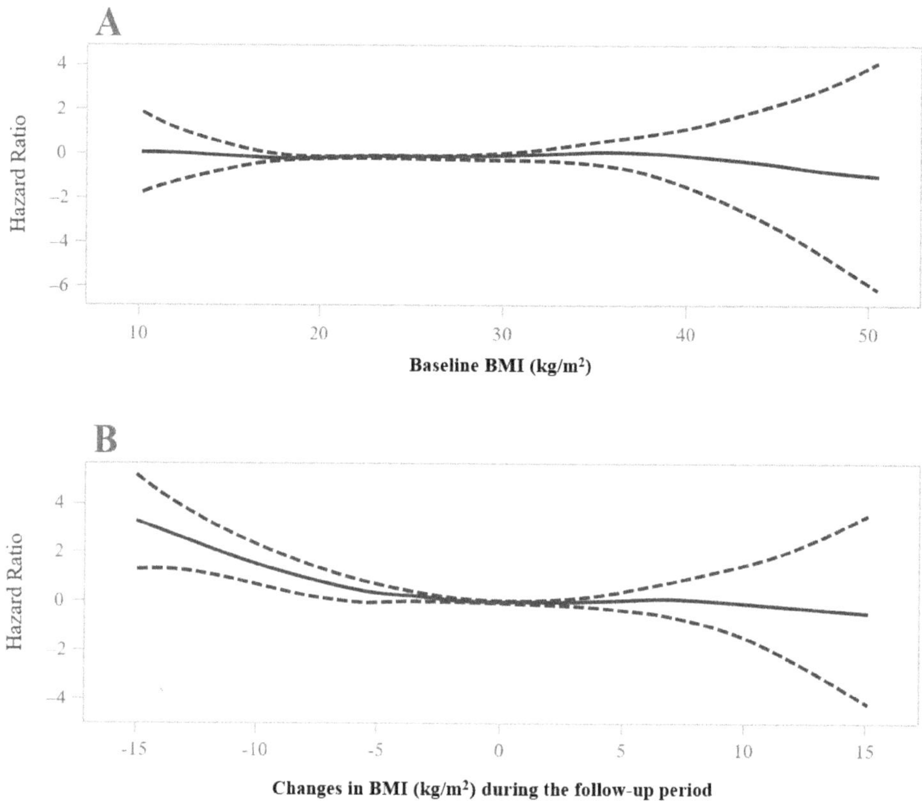

Figure 2. Cox proportional hazard spline curves showing associations between recurrent and persistent hematuria in glomerular disease and (**A**) baseline BMI (kg/m^2) and (**B**) changes in BMI (kg/m^2) during the follow-up period. BMI, body mass index.

Table 3 shows the independent relationship between BMI change quartiles and incident recurrent and persistent hematuria in glomerular disease, presented as HRs and 95% CIs. Compared to Q3 (0–3.59%), HRs (95% CI) for incident recurrent and persistent hematuria in glomerular disease were 1.204 (1.017–1.427) in Q1, 1.139 (0.955–1.360) in Q2, and 1.056 (0.887–1.257) in Q4. After adjusting for age, sex, smoking, alcohol drinking, physical activity, hypertension, diabetes, and dyslipidemia, the significant results were attenuated (Q1 (<−3.33%) vs. Q3 (0–3.59%); HR and 95% CI = 1.147 (0.968–1.359). Compared to the stable weight group (−10–10%), the HRs (95% CI) for incident recurrent and persistent hematuria in glomerular disease were 1.364 (1.029–1.808) and 0.985 (0.733–1.325) in the weight loss (<−10%) and gain groups (≥10%), respectively. The model was adjusted for the same confounders, and a significant association between weight loss and incident recurrent and persistent hematuria was observed. Figure 2B shows a spline curve for incident recurrent and persistent hematuria in glomerular disease according to BMI changes. Greater weight loss was linearly associated with incident recurrent and persistent hematuria in glomerular disease.

Table 3. Hazard ratios (HRs) and 95% confidence intervals (CIs) for the incidence of recurrent and persistent hematuria in glomerular disease according to body mass index (BMI) changes during the follow-up period.

	Body Mass Index Changes			
	Q1 (<−3.33%)	**Q2 (−3.33–0%)**	**Q3 (0–3.59%)**	**Q4 (≥3.59%)**
Total No.	87,100	76,762	97,384	87,051
Event	275	233	261	246
Person-years	991,691.5	881,718.5	1,122,379.1	1,002,816.5
IR (per 1000)	0.28	0.26	0.23	0.25
Crude HR	1.204 (1.017–1.427)	1.139 (0.955–1.360)	1.00 (reference)	1.056 (0.887–1.257)
Age- and sex-adjusted HR	1.148 (1.001–1.361)	1.124 (0.942–1.341)	1.00 (reference)	1.046 (0.879–1.245)
Fully adjusted HR	1.147 (0.968–1.359)	1.123 (0.941–1.341)	1.00 (reference)	1.051 (0.883–1.251)

	Body mass index changes		
	<−10%	−10.0–10%	≥10%
Total No.	13,759	318,304	16,234
Event	51	918	46
Person-years	153,186.61	3,659,063.74	186,355.18
IR (per 1000)	0.33	0.25	0.25
Crude HR	1.364 (1.029–1.808)	1.00 (reference)	0.985 (0.733–1.325)
Age- and sex-adjusted HR	1.246 (1.006–1.653)	1.00 (reference)	0.960 (0.714–1.290)
Fully adjusted HR	1.247 (1.001–1.655)	1.00 (reference)	0.967 (0.939–1.655)

BMI, body mass index; IR, incident rate; HR, hazard ratio; 95% CI, 95% confidence interval. Fully adjusted model: adjusted for age, sex, smoking, alcohol drinking, physical activity, hypertension, diabetes, and dyslipidemia.

4. Discussion

Although hematuria has been considered a representative symptom of renal disease, its role in the progression of kidney disease has received less attention than that given to proteinuria [22]. Recent studies have suggested that glomerular hematuria has a pathological role in promoting acute kidney injury (AKI) and progression to CKD through its nephrotoxic action of hemoglobin, heme inflammation, and oxidative stress [22,23]. Several epidemiological studies have reported that persistent hematuria is associated with an increased risk of renal function decline and ESRD during long follow-up periods [5,24,25]. Considering the important clinical implications of hematuria, it is important to investigate the effects of BMI on recurrent and persistent hematuria in glomerular disease. However, there are still conflicting results about the association between BMI and glomerular hematuria. Further large-scale epidemiologic studies are required to clarify the association between BMI and the incidence of recurrent and persistent hematuria in glomerular disease.

This study investigated the association between BMI and recurrent and persistent hematuria in glomerular disease diagnosed with ICD-10 codes recorded directly by clinicians using the large, population-based Korean National Health Insurance Service-National Health Screening Cohort. This is the first study to investigate the null association between BMI and recurrent and persistent hematuria in glomerular disease using a large-scale cohort. Particularly, it was found that weight loss greater than 10% was associated with recurrent and persistent hematuria.

Experimental evidence suggests that obesity has a role in the formation and progression of some glomerular lesions [26,27], but data for human glomerulonephritis are still insufficient. Previous studies have shown that a BMI $\geq$25 kg/m^2 was a risk factor for IgAN progression [28,29]. A study with 43 IgAN patients reported that a BMI $\geq$25 kg/m^2 was a significant predictor of disease progression [28]. Another study with 193 Japanese IgAN patients showed that even a slightly high BMI is a risk factor for disease progression [29]. In a recent cross-sectional study with 537 patients [30], the obese group was significantly associated with higher mesangial matrix expansion scores compared to the normal weight/overweight group (p = 0.020). In a cohort of 331 patients with biopsy-proven IgAN [17], patients with BMI greater than 25 kg/m^2 had worse clinical outcomes; however, there was no direct association between BMI and IgA progression. The studies were conducted on patients who had pre-existing IgAN, while this study investigated the effect of BMI on new-onset IgAN in the general population.

Unlike previous studies, this study found that BMI status was not associated with the incidence of recurrent and persistent hematuria in glomerular disease. In the current study, BMI was divided into four groups (<23 kg/m^2, 23–25 kg/m^2, 25–30 kg/m^2, and $\geq$30 kg/m^2). There was no difference in the results when further analysis was conducted by dividing the BMI into various criteria, such as BMI 18.5 kg/m^2 (cut-off). One of the possible reasons was the attributes of BMI. Traditionally, BMI is an indicator of obesity, but this study was unable to distinguish between body fat and muscle mass [31]. Additionally, BMI could not represent regional fat distribution. Further, obesity itself may affect the prevalence of glomerulopathy [32], exacerbating IgAN that has already occurred; however, obesity may have no impact on the incidence of hematuria in glomerular disease. More studies are needed using other indicators, such as body fat and waist circumference. In the current study, data on waist circumference were missing, and, therefore, it was excluded from further analysis.

Although BMI has limitations in indicating body components, it is commonly used as a marker in the assessment of nutritional status [33]. Several studies have reported the obesity paradox in populations with chronic heart failure [34], chronic obstructive pulmonary disease [35], and CKD [36,37]. The obesity paradox is likely to be explained by the fact that weight loss and physical frailty are associated with mortality in patients with chronic heart failure, chronic lung disease, and CKD [37]. The Chronic Renal Insufficiency Cohort Study, a multicenter prospective cohort study, showed that weight loss was associated with a 54% higher risk of death after dialysis therapy initiation in the stable weight group [16]. Ouyang et al. [15] showed that the incidence of ESRD in the underweight (<18.5 kg/m^2) group was higher than that in other BMI groups during a 47.1-month follow-up period. Unintentional weight loss, which might reflect nutritional deficit, has been reported as being associated with the progression of CKD [38]. Similar results were observed in the current study. This study found that the reduced BMI group (Q1 <−3.33% during the follow-up period) was associated with an increased risk of recurrent and persistent hematuria in glomerular disease. This association was attenuated after adjusting for confounding variables. However, interestingly, significant weight loss (greater than 10% during the follow-up period) was associated with an increased risk of recurrent and persistent hematuria in glomerular disease. The result remained significant even after adjusting for the same confounders.

This study has several limitations. First, the major limitation was that renal biopsy results were unobtainable. Since data from the NHIS-HEALS were used, recurrent and persistent hematuria in glomerular disease was defined using ICD-10 codes (N02.0–N02.8). Therefore, it was not possible to determine whether physicians recorded diagnostic codes based on renal biopsy results. According to a previous study conducted in Korea, among patients with asymptomatic isolated microscopic hematuria, IgAN was the most common cause, followed by idiopathic mesangial proliferative glomerulonephritis, with prevalence rates of 46.9% and 43.1%, respectively. IgAN, the most common cause of recurrent hematuria, is usually recorded in young adults during school urine screening tests [7]. However, the participants from NHIS-HEALS were middle-aged and older adults. Therefore, the incidence of IgAN could be lower than that previously reported [39]. Second, diseases commonly associated with recurrent hematuria, such as inflammatory conditions of the urethra, bladder, and prostate and malignancies that developed during the follow-up period, were not completely ruled out. Third, although we found that weight loss was associated with the incidence of recurrent and persistent hematuria, we could not determine the intentionality of weight loss in the cohort study. Unintentional weight loss is an involuntary decline in body weight over time and could reflect chronic diseases, psychological factors, social conditions, and undiagnosed illnesses [40]. In addition, only the association between BMI changes within 6 years and incident recurrent and persistent hematuria in glomerular disease was observed. Annual BMI changes could be a better predictor for incident recurrent and persistent hematuria in glomerular disease. Fourth, adiposity itself, directly and indirectly, affects the kidney through its endocrine activity, such as the production of adiponectin, leptin, and other inflammatory cytokines [5]. However, BMI could not fully reflect the amount of adiposity because the definition of BMI did not distinguish muscle from fat mass. Finally, this study included middle-aged and older Korean adults; therefore, there could have been a selection bias. Therefore, the results from this study cannot be generalized to other races/ethnicities. Further research is required to establish the association between body weight and recurrent and persistent hematuria in glomerular disease by considering the body composition data for young adults and annual changes in BMI. Finally, angiotensin-converting enzyme inhibitors/angiotensin receptor blockers are widely used in hypertension and kidney disease. However, the effect of these drugs could not be determined. Despite these weaknesses, this is the first study to investigate the impact of BMI and BMI changes on recurrent and persistent hematuria in glomerular disease using large-scale, population-based data. Although the results based on renal biopsy could not be determined, ICD-10 codes were used, which the physicians directly coded during the medical care process.

5. Conclusions

Baseline BMI was not associated with the incidence of recurrent and persistent hematuria in glomerular disease. Significant weight loss greater than 10% was associated with the incidence of recurrent and persistent hematuria in glomerular disease. Maintaining individuals' BMI could be a preventive strategy for the incidence of recurrent and persistent hematuria in glomerular disease in middle-aged and older Korean adults. Moreover, studies based on renal biopsy are required to determine these associations.

Supplementary Materials: The following supporting information can be downloaded at: https://www.mdpi.com/article/10.3390/biomedicines11030989/s1, Supplementary Figure S1. Flow chart of patients who have data follow-up data for BMI within 6 years.

Author Contributions: Y.-J.K. and J.E.L. contributed to the conception and design of the study, draft preparation, and article revision; M.K. and H.K., contributed to the conception and design of the study and data analysis. All authors have read and agreed to the published version of the manuscript.

Funding: This work was supported by the Korea Institute of Planning and Evaluation for Technology in Food, Agriculture and Forestry (IPET) through the High Value-added Food Technology Development Program funded by the Ministry of Agriculture, Food and Rural Affairs (MAFRA) (321030051HD030).

Institutional Review Board Statement: The Institutional Review Board (IRB) of Yongin Severance Hospital approved the present study (IRB No: 9-2020-0009).

Informed Consent Statement: Written informed consent has been obtained from the patient(s) to publish this paper.

Data Availability Statement: The data presented in this study are openly available on the National Health Insurance Data Sharing Service homepage; http://nhiss.or.kr (accessed on 21 January 2021).

Acknowledgments: All authors thank to Young Su Joo and Hae-Ryong Yun who give scientific advice to this article.

Conflicts of Interest: The authors declare no conflict of interest.

References

1. Hicks, J.; Mierau, G.; Wartchow, E.; Eldin, K. Renal diseases associated with hematuria in children and adolescents: A brief tutorial. *Ultrastruct. Pathol.* **2012**, *36*, 1–18. [CrossRef]
2. Yuste, C.; Gutierrez, E.; Sevillano, A.M.; Rubio-Navarro, A.; Amaro-Villalobos, J.M.; Ortiz, A.; Egido, J.; Praga, M.; Moreno, J.A. Pathogenesis of glomerular haematuria. *World J. Nephrol.* **2015**, *4*, 185–195. [CrossRef] [PubMed]

3. Moreno, J.A.; Sevillano, Á.; Gutiérrez, E.; Guerrero-Hue, M.; Vázquez-Carballo, C.; Yuste, C.; Herencia, C.; García-Caballero, C.; Praga, M.; Egido, J. Glomerular hematuria: Cause or consequence of renal inflammation? *Int. J. Mol. Sci.* **2019**, *20*, 2205. [CrossRef]
4. Kwon, H.; Lee, D.G.; Kang, H.C.; Lee, J.H. Incidence of isolated dipstick hematuria and its association with the glomerular filtration rate: A cross-sectional study from the korean national health and nutrition examination survey v (2010–2012). *Int. Urol. Nephrol.* **2016**, *48*, 451–456. [CrossRef] [PubMed]
5. Vivante, A.; Afek, A.; Frenkel-Nir, Y.; Tzur, D.; Farfel, A.; Golan, E.; Chaiter, Y.; Shohat, T.; Skorecki, K.; Calderon-Margalit, R. Persistent asymptomatic isolated microscopic hematuria in israeli adolescents and young adults and risk for end-stage renal disease. *JAMA* **2011**, *306*, 729–736. [CrossRef] [PubMed]
6. Coppo, R.; Fervenza, F.C. Persistent microscopic hematuria as a risk factor for progression of iga nephropathy: New floodlight on a nearly forgotten biomarker. *J. Am. Soc. Nephrol.* **2017**, *28*, 2831–2834. [CrossRef] [PubMed]
7. Park, Y.H.; Choi, J.Y.; Chung, H.S.; Koo, J.W.; Kim, S.Y.; Namgoong, M.K.; Park, Y.S.; Yoo, K.H.; Lee, K.Y.; Lee, D.Y.; et al. Hematuria and proteinuria in a mass school urine screening test. *Pediatr. Nephrol.* **2005**, *20*, 1126–1130. [CrossRef]
8. Tanaka, M.; Yamada, S.; Iwasaki, Y.; Sugishita, T.; Yonemoto, S.; Tsukamoto, T.; Fukui, S.; Takasu, K.; Muso, E. Impact of obesity on iga nephropathy: Comparative ultrastructural study between obese and non-obese patients. *Nephron Clin. Pract.* **2009**, *112*, c71–c78. [CrossRef] [PubMed]
9. Kovesdy, C.P.; Furth, S.L.; Zoccali, C. Obesity and kidney disease: Hidden consequences of the epidemic. *Can. J. Kidney Health Dis.* **2017**, *4*, 2054358117698669. [CrossRef]
10. Podkowińska, A.; Formanowicz, D. Chronic kidney disease as oxidative stress- and inflammatory-mediated cardiovascular disease. *Antioxidants* **2020**, *9*, 752. [CrossRef] [PubMed]
11. Tsuboi, N.; Utsunomiya, Y.; Kanzaki, G.; Koike, K.; Ikegami, M.; Kawamura, T.; Hosoya, T. Low glomerular density with glomerulomegaly in obesity-related glomerulopathy. *Clin. J. Am. Soc. Nephrol.* **2012**, *7*, 735–741. [CrossRef] [PubMed]
12. Alicic, R.Z.; Patakoti, R.; Tuttle, K.R. Direct and indirect effects of obesity on the kidney. *Adv. Chronic Kidney Dis.* **2013**, *20*, 121–127. [CrossRef] [PubMed]
13. Kittiskulnam, P.; Kanjanabuch, T.; Tangmanjitjaroen, K.; Chancharoenthana, W.; Praditpornsilpa, K.; Eiam-Ong, S. The beneficial effects of weight reduction in overweight patients with chronic proteinuric immunoglobulin a nephropathy: A randomized controlled trial. *J. Ren. Nutr.* **2014**, *24*, 200–207. [CrossRef] [PubMed]
14. Afshinnia, F.; Wilt, T.J.; Duval, S.; Esmaeili, A.; Ibrahim, H.N. Weight loss and proteinuria: Systematic review of clinical trials and comparative cohorts. *Nephrol. Dial. Transplant.* **2010**, *25*, 1173–1183. [CrossRef]
15. Ouyang, Y.; Xie, J.; Yang, M.; Zhang, X.; Ren, H.; Wang, W.; Chen, N. Underweight is an independent risk factor for renal function deterioration in patients with iga nephropathy. *PLoS ONE* **2016**, *11*, e0162044. [CrossRef]
16. Ku, E.; Kopple, J.D.; Johansen, K.L.; McCulloch, C.E.; Go, A.S.; Xie, D.; Lin, F.; Hamm, L.L.; He, J.; Kusek, J.W.; et al. Longitudinal weight change during ckd progression and its association with subsequent mortality. *Am. J. Kidney Dis.* **2018**, *71*, 657–665. [CrossRef]
17. Berthoux, F.; Mariat, C.; Maillard, N. Overweight/obesity revisited as a predictive risk factor in primary iga nephropathy. *Nephrol. Dial. Transplant.* **2013**, *28* (Suppl. S4), iv160–iv166. [CrossRef]
18. Nagaraju, S.P.; Rangaswamy, D.; Mareddy, A.S.; Prasad, S.; Kaza, S.; Shenoy, S.; Saraf, K.; Attur, R.P.; Parthasarathy, R.; Kosuru, S.; et al. Impact of body mass index on progression of primary immunoglobulin a nephropathy. *Saudi J. Kidney Dis. Transpl.* **2018**, *29*, 318–325. [CrossRef]
19. Wu, C.; Wang, A.Y.; Li, G.; Wang, L. Association of high body mass index with development of interstitial fibrosis in patients with iga nephropathy. *BMC Nephrol.* **2018**, *19*, 381. [CrossRef]
20. Seong, S.C.; Kim, Y.Y.; Park, S.K.; Khang, Y.H.; Kim, H.C.; Park, J.H.; Kang, H.J.; Do, C.H.; Song, J.S.; Lee, E.J.; et al. Cohort profile: The national health insurance service-national health screening cohort (nhis-heals) in korea. *BMJ Open.* **2017**, *7*, e016640. [CrossRef]
21. Seo, M.H.; Lee, W.Y.; Kim, S.S.; Kang, J.H.; Kang, J.H.; Kim, K.K.; Kim, B.Y.; Kim, Y.H.; Kim, W.J.; Kim, E.M.; et al. 2018 korean society for the study of obesity guideline for the management of obesity in korea. *J. Obes. Metab. Syndr.* **2019**, *28*, 40–45. [CrossRef]
22. Orlandi, P.F.; Fujii, N.; Roy, J.; Chen, H.Y.; Lee Hamm, L.; Sondheimer, J.H.; He, J.; Fischer, M.J.; Rincon-Choles, H.; Krishnan, G.; et al. Hematuria as a risk factor for progression of chronic kidney disease and death: Findings from the chronic renal insufficiency cohort (cric) study. *BMC Nephrol.* **2018**, *19*, 150. [CrossRef] [PubMed]
23. Moreno, J.A.; Yuste, C.; Gutiérrez, E.; Sevillano, Á.M.; Rubio-Navarro, A.; Amaro-Villalobos, J.M.; Praga, M.; Egido, J. Haematuria as a risk factor for chronic kidney disease progression in glomerular diseases: A review. *Pediatr. Nephrol.* **2016**, *31*, 523–533. [CrossRef]
24. Goto, M.; Wakai, K.; Kawamura, T.; Ando, M.; Endoh, M.; Tomino, Y. A scoring system to predict renal outcome in iga nephropathy: A nationwide 10-year prospective cohort study. *Nephrol. Dial. Transplant.* **2009**, *24*, 3068–3074. [CrossRef] [PubMed]
25. Sevillano, A.M.; Gutiérrez, E.; Yuste, C.; Cavero, T.; Mérida, E.; Rodríguez, P.; García, A.; Morales, E.; Fernández, C.; Martínez, M.A.; et al. Remission of hematuria improves renal survival in iga nephropathy. *J. Am. Soc. Nephrol.* **2017**, *28*, 3089–3099. [CrossRef]
26. Ribstein, J.; du Cailar, G.; Mimran, A. Combined renal effects of overweight and hypertension. *Hypertension* **1995**, *26*, 610–615. [CrossRef] [PubMed]

27. Verani, R.R. Obesity-associated focal segmental glomerulosclerosis: Pathological features of the lesion and relationship with cardiomegaly and hyperlipidemia. *Am. J. Kidney Dis.* **1992**, *20*, 629–634. [CrossRef] [PubMed]
28. Kataoka, H.; Ohara, M.; Shibui, K.; Sato, M.; Suzuki, T.; Amemiya, N.; Watanabe, Y.; Honda, K.; Mochizuki, T.; Nitta, K. Overweight and obesity accelerate the progression of iga nephropathy: Prognostic utility of a combination of bmi and histopathological parameters. *Clin. Exp. Nephrol.* **2012**, *16*, 706–712. [CrossRef] [PubMed]
29. Shimamoto, M.; Ohsawa, I.; Suzuki, H.; Hisada, A.; Nagamachi, S.; Honda, D.; Inoshita, H.; Shimizu, Y.; Horikoshi, S.; Tomino, Y. Impact of body mass index on progression of iga nephropathy among japanese patients. *J. Clin. Lab. Anal.* **2015**, *29*, 353–360. [CrossRef]
30. Hong, Y.A.; Min, J.W.; Ha, M.A.; Koh, E.S.; Kim, H.D.; Ban, T.H.; Kim, Y.S.; Kim, Y.K.; Kim, D.; Shin, S.J.; et al. The impact of obesity on the severity of clinicopathologic parameters in patients with iga nephropathy. *J. Clin. Med.* **2020**, *9*, 2824. [CrossRef]
31. Nuttall, F.Q. Body mass index: Obesity, bmi, and health: A critical review. *Nutr. Today* **2015**, *50*, 117–128. [CrossRef]
32. D'Agati, V.D.; Chagnac, A.; de Vries, A.P.; Levi, M.; Porrini, E.; Herman-Edelstein, M.; Praga, M. Obesity-related glomerulopathy: Clinical and pathologic characteristics and pathogenesis. *Nat. Rev. Nephrol.* **2016**, *12*, 453–471. [CrossRef] [PubMed]
33. Bailey, K.; Ferro-Luzzi, A. Use of body mass index of adults in assessing individual and community nutritional status. *Bull. World Health Organ.* **1995**, *73*, 673. [PubMed]
34. Oreopoulos, A.; Padwal, R.; Kalantar-Zadeh, K.; Fonarow, G.C.; Norris, C.M.; McAlister, F.A. Body mass index and mortality in heart failure: A meta-analysis. *Am. Heart J.* **2008**, *156*, 13–22. [CrossRef] [PubMed]
35. Prescott, E.; Almdal, T.; Mikkelsen, K.L.; Tofteng, C.L.; Vestbo, J.; Lange, P. Prognostic value of weight change in chronic obstructive pulmonary disease: Results from the copenhagen city heart study. *Eur. Respir. J.* **2002**, *20*, 539–544. [CrossRef]
36. Schmidt, D.; Salahudeen, A. The obesity-survival paradox in hemodialysis patients: Why do overweight hemodialysis patients live longer? *Nutr. Clin. Pract.* **2007**, *22*, 11–15. [CrossRef] [PubMed]
37. Hainer, V.; Aldhoon-Hainerová, I. Obesity paradox does exist. *Diabetes Care* **2013**, *36* (Suppl. S2), S276–S281. [CrossRef] [PubMed]
38. Ku, E.; Kopple, J.D.; McCulloch, C.E.; Warady, B.A.; Furth, S.L.; Mak, R.H.; Grimes, B.A.; Mitsnefes, M. Associations between weight loss, kidney function decline, and risk of esrd in the chronic kidney disease in children (ckid) cohort study. *Am. J. Kidney Dis.* **2018**, *71*, 648–656. [CrossRef]
39. Schena, F.P.; Nistor, I. Epidemiology of iga nephropathy: A global perspective. *Semin. Nephrol.* **2018**, *38*, 435–442. [CrossRef] [PubMed]
40. Alibhai, S.M.; Greenwood, C.; Payette, H. An approach to the management of unintentional weight loss in elderly people. *CMAJ* **2005**, *172*, 773–780. [CrossRef]

biomedicines

MDPI

Article

Single Nucleotide Polymorphisms of the *RAC1* Gene as Novel Susceptibility Markers for Neuropathy and Microvascular Complications in Type 2 Diabetes

Iuliia Azarova [1,2], Elena Klyosova [2,3] and Alexey Polonikov [3,4,*]

[1] Department of Biological Chemistry, Kursk State Medical University, 3 Karl Marx Street, Kursk 305041, Russia; azzzzar@yandex.ru or azarovaje@kursksmu.net

[2] Laboratory of Biochemical Genetics and Metabolomics, Research Institute for Genetic and Molecular Epidemiology, Kursk State Medical University, 18 Yamskaya St., Kursk 305041, Russia; ecless@yandex.ru or klesovaeu@kursksmu.net

[3] Department of Biology, Medical Genetics and Ecology, Kursk State Medical University, 3 Karl Marx Street, Kursk 305041, Russia

[4] Laboratory of Statistical Genetics and Bioinformatics, Research Institute for Genetic and Molecular Epidemiology, Kursk State Medical University, 18 Yamskaya St., Kursk 305041, Russia

* Correspondence: polonikov@rambler.ru or polonikovav@kursksmu.net

Abstract: Single nucleotide polymorphisms (SNP) in the *RAC1* (Rac family small GTPase 1) gene have recently been linked to type 2 diabetes (T2D) and hyperglycemia due to their contribution to impaired redox homeostasis. The present study was designed to determine whether the common SNPs of the *RAC1* gene are associated with diabetic complications such as neuropathy (DN), retinopathy (DR), nephropathy, angiopathy of the lower extremities (DA), and diabetic foot syndrome. A total of 1470 DNA samples from T2D patients were genotyped for six common SNPs by the MassArray Analyzer-4 system. The genotype rs7784465-T/C of *RAC1* was associated with an increased risk of DR ($p = 0.016$) and DA ($p = 0.03$) in males, as well as with DR in females ($p = 0.01$). Furthermore, the SNP rs836478 showed an association with DR ($p = 0.005$) and DN ($p = 0.025$) in males, whereas the SNP rs10238136 was associated with DA in females ($p = 0.002$). In total, three *RAC1* haplotypes showed significant associations (FDR < 0.05) with T2D complications in a sex-specific manner. The study's findings demonstrate, for the first time, that the *RAC1* gene's polymorphisms represent novel and sex-specific markers of neuropathy and microvascular complications in type 2 diabetes, and that the gene could be a new target for the pharmacological inhibition of oxidative stress as a means of preventing diabetic complications.

Keywords: Rac family small GTPase 1 (RAC1); type 2 diabetes mellitus; diabetic neuropathy; diabetic retinopathy; diabetic nephropathy; diabetic angiopathy of the lower extremities; diabetic foot syndrome

1. Introduction

Over 500 million people worldwide are affected by type 2 diabetes (T2D), which, along with obesity, is the second most frequent endocrinological disease [1]. About 7.8 million people in the Russian Federation have diabetes, with T2D accounting for the majority of cases [1]. Type 2 diabetes is associated with a multitude of disorders in lipid, protein, nucleotide metabolism, and redox homeostasis, leading to long-term complications that made T2D the ninth cause of mortality in 2020 [2]. In particular, impaired redox homeostasis is thought to be an important pathological condition underlying oxidative stress that contributes to the initiation and progression of type 2 diabetes [3–5]. Hyperglycemia, an increase in reactive oxygen species (ROS) production with cytosolic NADPH oxidase, and a deficiency in key antioxidants such as reduced glutathione (GSH) are considered to be the major damaging factors that are responsible for the structural and functional alterations in the retina, kidneys, nerves, and vessels in diabetics that ultimately lead to complications such as diabetic retinopathy (DR), diabetic nephropathy (DF), diabetic neuropathy (DN), diabetic angiopathy of the lower extremities (DA), and diabetic foot syndrome (DFS) [6–9].

The NADPH oxidase (NOX) enzyme is primarily responsible for the generation of superoxide anion radicals, which accumulate excessively in the cell and cause oxidative stress [10]. Once generated, these superoxides are rapidly dismutated into hydrogen peroxide, either spontaneously or via superoxide dismutase [11]. Other ROS are generated through the reactions of the superoxide radical with nitric oxide to form peroxynitrite, the peroxidase-catalyzed formation of hypochlorous acid from hydrogen peroxide, and the iron-catalyzed Fenton's reaction which produces hydroxyl radicals [12,13]. Notably, increased ROS generation was found to interact with the proteins of the insulin signaling pathway, contributing to insulin resistance [14,15] and triggering the dysfunction and apoptosis of pancreatic beta-cells [16].

The NOX enzyme represents a multi-subunit complex consisting of several proteins, among which small GTPases, such as RAC1 and RAC2, are known to activate the holoenzyme [17]. A total of two experimental studies [18,19] have shown that the transcriptional activation of the *RAC1* gene in diabetic mice has been found to contribute to mitochondrial damage and retinopathy, suggesting at least a causal role of this gene in diabetic complications. We have recently observed that the single nucleotide polymorphisms (SNP) of the *RAC1* gene are tightly associated with impaired redox homeostasis, an increased risk of type 2 diabetes, and hyperglycemia [20]. Pursuing further interests in the role of this gene within T2D, the purpose of the present study was to investigate whether the polymorphisms of the *RAC1* gene contribute to the development of common diabetic complications, such as retinopathy, nephropathy, neuropathy, angiopathy of the lower extremities, and diabetic foot syndrome.

2. Materials and Methods

2.1. Study Participants and Diagnosis of Type 2 Diabetes

The Regional Ethics Review Committee of Kursk State Medical University gave its approval to the study protocol, which complied with the ethical standards of the Declaration of Helsinki. Before being enrolled in the study, each subject provided their written informed consent. A total of 1470 patients with type 2 diabetes were included in the study. Most of the study participants were Russians from the Kursk region (central Russia). All were patients that had been admitted to the Endocrinology Division of the Kursk Emergency Hospital between November 2016 and October 2019. The following WHO criteria [21,22] were used to verify the T2D diagnosis: a fasting blood glucose (FBG) level of $\geq$7.0 mmol/L, a random blood glucose level of $\geq$11.1 mmol/L, and/or a glycated hemoglobin (HbA1c) level of $\geq$6.5%. The criteria for the inclusion of T2D patients in the study were: (1) a physician-verified diagnosis of T2D, confirmed by clinical, laboratory, and instrumental investigations; (2) an age of over 35 years old; and (3) written informed consent to participate in the study. The criteria for excluding patients from the study were the following: (1) an age of less than 35 years; (2) an absence of written informed consent to participate in the study; and (3) advanced-stage diabetes or the decompensation of diabetes, diabetic coma, immune-mediated or idiopathic type 1 diabetes, gestational diabetes, MODY types of diabetes, diseases of the exocrine pancreas, such as pancreatitis, pancreatic trauma, or pancreatectomy, pancreatic tumors, hereditary diseases affecting the pancreas, or any other endocrine disorders. All of the study's participants completed a questionnaire [23] on the risk factors of type 2 diabetes.

2.2. Genetic Analysis

Fasted venous blood samples were collected from all the study participants, and the genomic DNA was purified by a spin column QIAamp Blood Mini Kit with the use of a robotic workstation QiaCube (QIAGEN, Germany). In total, six commonly tagged SNPs of the *RAC1* gene, such as rs4724800, rs7784465, rs10951982, rs10238136, rs836478, and rs9374, were selected for the study, as described previously [20]. The SNP genotyping was performed using MALDI-TOF mass spectrometry with the MassArray-4 System (Agena Bioscience Inc., San Diego, CA, USA). The primer sequences that were used for the genotyping are available upon request. The genotyping analysis was performed blindly, with regard to the case–control status to ensure quality control. Repeat genotyping was performed on approximately 10% of the samples, randomly selected from the T2D group, and the repeatability test yielded a 100% concordance rate.

2.3. Biochemical Analysis

All the biochemical investigations were performed using fasted whole blood samples that were collected in standard sterile tubes with lithium heparin, and immediately centrifuged at 3500 rpm, according to the manufacturer's instructions (Cell Biolabs, San Diego, CA, USA; Abcam, Waltham, MA, USA). The plasma samples were aliquoted and stored at −80 °C until their further use. For the determination of oxidized glutathione (GSSG), the plasma was immediately deproteinized with trichloroacetic acid. The plasma hydrogen peroxide levels were assessed in 489 T2D patients, whereas the GSSG levels were measured in 258 diabetics that were recruited at the final study phase (between March 2019 and October 2019). The GSSG levels were determined by a fluorometric assay protocol (GSH/GSSG Ratio Detection Assay Kit II, Abcam, Waltham, MA, USA) that used a proprietary, non-fluorescent, water-soluble dye that became strongly fluorescent upon reacting with GSH. The levels of ROS were quantified by fluorometric assay using the OxiSelect™ In Vitro ROS/RNS Assay Kit (Cell Biolabs, San Diego, CA, USA), which employed a proprietary quenched fluorogenic probe, dichlorodihydrofluorescin DiOxyQ (DCFH-DiOxyQ), which is a specific ROS/RNS probe. It was first primed with a quench removal reagent and subsequently stabilized in a highly reactive DCFH form. In this reactive state, the ROS and RNS species react with the DCFH, which is rapidly oxidized to the highly fluorescent 2′,7′-dichlorodihydrofluorescein. The standard curve of H_2O_2 was used to quantify the ROS concentrations in the plasma samples. Absorbance at 405 nm and fluorescence at 480 nm excitation/530 nm emission were measured on a microplate reader Varioscan Flash (Thermo Fisher Scientific, Waltham, MA, USA). The concentrations of glycated hemoglobin, the fasting blood glucose in blood plasma were determined with the use of a semi-automatic biochemical analyzer Clima MC-15 (Ral Tecnica para el Laboratorio, S.A., Barcelona, Spain) and the reagents produced by DIAKON-DS, Moscow, (Russia). These biochemical and genetic analyses were performed at the Research Institute for Genetic and Molecular Epidemiology of Kursk State Medical University, Kursk (Russia).

2.4. Statistical and Bioinformatics Analysis

Statistical power was estimated using the genetic association study power calculator (http://csg.sph.umich.edu/abecasis/gas_power_calculator/, accessed on 12 June 2016). Based on the sample size of 1470 people with T2D, a sub-group association analysis of the *RAC1* polymorphisms with diabetic complications could detect a genotype relative risk of 1.25–1.50, assuming a 79.1–90.0% power and a 5% type I error (0.05). The chi-square test was used to compare the genotype frequencies in T2D patients to the values predicted by the Hardy–Weinberg equilibrium assumption. The association between the *RAC1* gene polymorphisms and diabetic combinations was evaluated by a multiple logistic regression analysis, with the calculation of odds ratios (OR) and 95% confidence intervals (95%CI) adjusted for age, sex, and body mass index (BMI). The associations were analyzed using the SNPStats software [24]. A codominant model was used to present the results in tables. A p-value of $\leq$0.05 was selected as statistically significant. To control for the multiple testing of the SNP-phenotype associations, the calculated p-values were adjusted by the false discovery rate (FDR). A Q-value of $\leq$0.05 was considered statistically significant to interpret the genotype–phenotype associations [25].

The Kolmogorov–Smirnov test was used to determine the normality of the biochemical parameters. Age and BMI were expressed as means with standard deviations and compared between the groups by the Student's *t*-test. The non-normally distributed traits (glycated hemoglobin, fasting blood glucose, hydrogen peroxide, and total glutathione) were expressed as medians with the first and third quartiles (Q1–Q3) and compared between the groups with the Kruskal–Wallis test. These statistical calculations were performed using the STATISTICA for Windows v13.0 package (TIBCO, Palo Alto, CA, USA).

3. Results

3.1. Demographic, Clinical and Laboratory Characteristics of Patients

The demographic, clinical, and laboratory characteristics of the study patients are shown in Table 1. The majority of the T2D patients had diabetic neuropathy (92.3%) and diabetic retinopathy (71.2%). Other T2D complications included diabetic angiopathy of the lower extremities (65.9%), diabetic nephropathy (38.4%), diabetic foot syndrome (7.6%), and coronary artery disease (32.5%). The patients with the above complications had a significantly longer duration of T2D ($p = 0.001$). As can be seen from Table 1, there were no regularities or trends in the quantitative parameters of redox homeostasis, such as glutathione or hydrogen peroxide, regardless of the type of diabetes complication.

Table 1. Demographic, clinical, and biochemical characteristics of the study patients.

Baseline Characteristics	T2D Patients (n = 1470)		*p*-Value *
	Without Complication	With Complication	
	Diabetic retinopathy		
Sample size, n (%)	407 (28.8)	1007 (71.2)	-
Age, mean ± SD	58.50 ± 11.73	62.99 ± 9.37	**<0.0001**
Males, n (%)	179 (44.0)	279 (27.7)	**<0.0001**
Females, n (%)	228 (56.0)	728 (72.3)	
Body mass index (kg/m^2), mean ± SD	31.65 ± 6.91	32.57 ± 6.55	0.18
Duration of diabetes, median (Q1;Q3)	2.0 (1.0; 8.0)	10.0 (6.0; 16.0)	**0.001**
HbA_{1C} (%), Me (Q1; Q3)	9.3 (7.9; 11.1)	9.0 (7.7; 10.6)	**0.033**
FBG (mmol/L), Me (Q1; Q3)	12.8 (10.3; 15.8)	12.0 (9.53; 15.0)	**0.001**
H_2O_2 (mmol/L), Me(Q1;Q3)	3.94 (2.70; 5.27)	3.66 (2.58; 4.92)	0.11
GSSG/GSH (mmol/L), Me(Q1;Q3)	2.70 (1.29; 3.90)	1.28 (0.50; 3.74)	**0.0036**
	Diabetic nephropathy		
Sample size, n (%)	887 (61.6)	553 (38.4)	-
Age, mean ± SD	58.86 ± 10.29	66.11 ± 8.60	**<0.0001**
Males, n (%)	379 (42.7)	101 (18.3)	**<0.0001**
Females, n (%)	507 (57.3)	452 (81.7)	
Body mass index (kg/m^2), mean ± SD	31.62 ± 6.88	33.15 ± 6.29	**<0.0001**
Duration of diabetes, median (Q1;Q3)	7.0 (2.0; 12.0)	11.0 (6.0; 17.0)	**<0.0001**
HbA_{1C} (%), Me (Q1; Q3)	9.0 (7.7; 10.5)	9.2 (7.8; 11.0)	0.09
FBG (mmol/L), Me (Q1; Q3)	12.0 (9.5; 15.0)	12.6 (10.0; 15.9)	**0.026**
H_2O_2 (mmol/L), Me(Q1;Q3)	3.73 (2.62; 5.09)	3.74 (2.66; 4.99)	0.93
GSSG/GSH (mmol/L), Me(Q1;Q3)	1.31 (0.56; 3.77)	1.99 (0.56; 3.90)	0.29
	Diabetic neuropathy		
Sample size, n (%)	109 (7.7)	1309 (92.3)	-
Age, mean ± SD	53.66 ± 12.99	62.37 ± 9.76	**<0.0001**
Males, n (%)	58 (53.21)	401 (30.63)	**<0.0001**
Females, n (%)	50 (46.79)	908 (69.37)	
Body mass index (kg/m^2), mean ± SD	29.30 ± 6.24	32.57 ± 6.63	**<0.0001**
Duration of diabetes, median (Q1;Q3)	1.0 (0.1; 1.0)	10.0 (4.0; 15.0)	**0.001**
HbA_{1C} (%), Me (Q1; Q3)	9.4 (7.7; 11.3)	9.0 (7.7; 10.8)	0.18
FBG (mmol/L), Me (Q1; Q3)	13.1 (10.0)	12.2 (9.8; 15.2)	0.14
H_2O_2 (mmol/L), Me(Q1;Q3)	3.98 (3.21; 6.41)	3.72 (2.6; 4.94)	**0.013**
GSSG/GSH (mmol/L), Me(Q1;Q3)	1.31 (0.29; 3.66)	1.64 (0.57; 3.80)	0.55

Table 1. *Cont.*

Baseline Characteristics	T2D Patients (n = 1470)		p-Value *
	Without Complication	With Complication	
	Angiopathy of the lower extremities		
Sample size, n (%)	502 (34.1)	968 (65.9)	-
Age, mean ± SD	58.33 ± 12.09	63.19 ± 9.27	**<0.0001**
Males, n (%)	210 (41.8)	272 (28.1)	**<0.0001**
Females, n (%)	291 (58.2)	696 (71.9)	
Body mass index (kg/m^2), mean ± SD	31.12 ± 6.51	32.81 ± 6.65	**<0.0001**
Duration of diabetes, median (Q1;Q3)	5.0 (1.0; 11.0)	10.0 (5.0; 15.0)	**<0.0001**
HbA$_{1C}$ (%), Me (Q1; Q3)	9.2 (7.75; 11.2)	9.0 (7.7; 10.5)	0.054
FBG (mmol/L), Me (Q1; Q3)	12.5 (9.7; 15.6)	12.0 (9.79; 15.0)	0.23
H_2O_2 (mmol/L), Me(Q1;Q3)	3.70 (2.76; 5.12)	3.72 (2.58; 5.02)	0.58
GSSG/GSH (mmol/L), Me(Q1;Q3)	1.35 (0.56; 3.82)	1.70 (0.51; 3.78)	0.66
	Diabetic foot syndrome		
Sample size, n (%)	1309 (92.4)	107 (7.6)	-
Age, mean ± SD	61.57 ± 10.45	63.35 ± 8.29	0.087
Males, n (%)	424 (32.4)	34 (31.8)	0.89
Females, n (%)	884 (67.6)	73 (68.2)	
Body mass index (kg/m^2), mean ± SD	32.27 ± 6.67	33.02 ± 6.65	0.26
Duration of diabetes, median (Q1;Q3)	9.0 (3.0; 14.0)	12.0 (6.0; 18.0)	**0.0002**
HbA$_{1C}$ (%), Me (Q1; Q3)	9.1 (7.7; 10.9)	8.4 (7.5; 10.0)	**0.032**
FBG (mmol/L), Me (Q1; Q3)	12.4 (9.88; 15.32)	10.9 (8.86; 14.3)	**0.012**
H_2O_2 (mmol/L), Me(Q1;Q3)	3.81 (2.73; 5.14)	2.72 (1.95; 4.03)	**0.0003**
GSSG/GSH (mmol/L), Me(Q1;Q3)	1.41 (0.51; 3.71)	2.83 (1.23; 3.98)	0.051

* Bold is statistically significant p-value.

3.2. Association of *RAC1* Gene Polymorphisms with Diabetic Retinopathy

The frequency of the minor allele rs7784465-C was significantly higher in the patients with DR within the entire group (OR 1.35, 95%CI 1.09–1.68, p = 0.006) and in males (OR 1.52, 95%CI 1.05–2.21, p = 0.032) after a sex-stratified analysis. The alternative allele rs836478-T was associated with DR in the entire group of patients with DR (OR 1.34, 95%CI 1.14–1.59, p = 0.0005), in males (OR 1.51, 95%CI 1.15–1.99, p = 0.003), and in females (OR 1.27, 95%CI 1.02–1.57, p = 0.03). The genotype frequencies of the studied SNPs in diabetics with and without DR are shown in Table 2.

Table 2. Genotype frequencies for the *RAC1* gene polymorphisms in T2D patients with and without diabetic retinopathy (DR).

SNP	Genotype	T2D Patients		P (Q) [1]	OR (95% CI) [2]
		Without DR n (%)	With DR n (%)		
		Entire Group			
rs4724800 A>G	A/A A/G G/G	253 (62.9) 127 (31.6) 22 (5.5)	581 (58.2) 370 (37.1) 47 (4.7)	0.14 (0.33)	1.00 1.28 (0.99–1.65) 0.93 (0.54–1.61)
rs7784465 T>C	T/T T/C C/C	280 (70.5) 104 (26.2) 13 (3.3)	618 (63.4) 317 (32.5) 40 (4.1)	**0.034** (0.15)	1.00 **1.36 (1.04–1.77)** 1.39 (0.72–2.69)
rs10951982 G>A	G/G G/A A/A	272 (67.5) 112 (27.8) 19 (4.7)	624 (62.6) 329 (33) 43 (4.3)	0.19 (0.38)	1.00 1.27 (0.98–1.66) 1.00 (0.56–1.79)
rs10238136 A>T	A/A A/T T/T	374 (95.2) 18 (4.6) 1 (0.2)	935 (94.2) 57 (5.7) 1 (0.1)	0.51 (0.55)	1.00 1.31 (0.75–2.28) 0.40 (0.02–6.43)
rs836478 C>T	C/C C/T T/T	144 (35.6) 194 (48) 66 (16.3)	278 (28.4) 469 (48) 231 (23.6)	**0.0013 (0.023)**	1.00 1.30 (0.99–1.70) **1.89 (1.33–2.69)**
rs9374 G>A	G/G G/A A/A	275 (67.6) 116 (28.5) 16 (3.9)	614 (63) 324 (33.3) 36 (3.7)	0.21 (0.38)	1.00 1.26 (0.97–1.64) 1.02 (0.54–1.92)

Table 2. *Cont.*

SNP	Genotype	T2D Patients: Without DR n (%)	T2D Patients: With DR n (%)	P (Q) [1]	OR (95% CI) [2]
Males					
rs4724800 A>G	A/A	111 (63.1)	163 (59.5)	0.42 (0.52)	1.00
	A/G	53 (30.1)	96 (35)		1.28 (0.84–1.97)
	G/G	12 (6.8)	15 (5.5)		0.84 (0.37–1.91)
rs7784465 T>C	T/T	129 (75.4)	167 (63)	**0.016** (0.096)	1.00
	T/C	37 (21.6)	92 (34.7)		**1.93 (1.22–3.06)**
	C/C	5 (2.9)	6 (2.3)		1.11 (0.32–3.83)
rs10951982 G>A	G/G	121 (68.4)	176 (63.8)	0.28 (0.46)	1.00
	G/A	44 (24.9)	87 (31.5)		1.37 (0.88–2.15)
	A/A	12 (6.8)	13 (4.7)		0.79 (0.34–1.86)
rs10238136 A>T	A/A	161 (94.7)	257 (93.1)	0.14 (0.34)	1.00
	A/T	8 (4.7)	19 (6.9)		1.67 (0.69–4.05)
	T/T	1 (0.6)	0 (0)		NA
rs836478 C>T	C/C	63 (35.4)	71 (26.4)	**0.0051 (0.046)**	1.00
	C/T	89 (50)	128 (47.6)		1.38 (0.88–2.18)
	T/T	26 (14.6)	70 (26)		**2.58 (1.43–4.63)**
rs9374 G>A	G/G	122 (68.2)	169 (62.8)	0.15 (0.34)	1.00
	G/A	46 (25.7)	90 (33.5)		1.43 (0.92–2.22)
	A/A	11 (6.2)	10 (3.7)		0.66 (0.26–1.67)
Females					
rs4724800 A>G	A/A	142 (62.8)	418 (57.7)	0.31 (0.47)	1.00
	A/G	74 (32.7)	274 (37.9)		1.28 (0.93–1.77)
	G/G	10 (4.4)	32 (4.4)		1.03 (0.49–2.17)
rs7784465 T>C	T/T	151 (66.8)	451 (63.5)	0.52 (0.55)	1.00
	T/C	67 (29.6)	225 (31.7)		1.12 (0.80–1.56)
	C/C	8 (3.5)	34 (4.8)		1.49 (0.67–3.32)
rs10951982 G>A	G/G	151 (66.8)	448 (62.2)	0.43 (0.52)	1.00
	G/A	68 (30.1)	242 (33.6)		1.22 (0.88–1.69)
	A/A	7 (3.1)	30 (4.2)		1.32 (0.56–3.09)
rs10238136 A>T	A/A	213 (95.5)	678 (94.6)	0.70 (0.70)	1.00
	A/T	10 (4.5)	38 (5.3)		1.14 (0.56–2.33)
	T/T	0 (0)	1 (0.1)		NA
rs836478 C>T	C/C	81 (35.8)	207 (29.2)	0.098 (0.34)	1.00
	C/T	105 (46.5)	341 (48.1)		1.28 (0.91–1.79)
	T/T	40 (17.7)	161 (22.7)		1.59 (1.03–2.46)
rs9374 G>A	G/G	153 (67.1)	445 (63.1)	0.40 (0.52)	1.00
	G/A	70 (30.7)	234 (33.2)		1.17 (0.85–1.63)
	A/A	5 (2.2)	26 (3.7)		1.65 (0.62–4.39)

[1] *p*-value (FDR-adjusted *p*-value) adjusted for age, sex, and BMI. [2] Odds ratio with 95% confidence intervals adjusted for age, sex, and BMI (codominant genetic model). Bold is statistically significant *P*- and *Q*-values.

The genotypes rs7784465-T/C and rs836478-T/T were associated with the risk of diabetic retinopathy in the entire group of diabetics. A sex-stratified association analysis showed that the polymorphisms rs7784465 and rs836478 were associated with an increased risk for DR in males, whereas in females, no difference in the genotype frequencies for these SNPs was seen between the patients with and without DR. The estimated frequencies of the *RAC1* haplotypes in T2D patients with and without DR are shown in Table 3.

Table 3. Estimated common haplotype frequencies of *RAC1* gene in T2D patients with and without diabetic retinopathy.

Haplotype Number	SNPs: rs4724800	rs7784465	rs10951982	rs10238136	rs836478	rs9374	T2D Patients: Without DR (Haplotype Frequency [1])	T2D Patients: With DR (Haplotype Frequency [1])	OR (95% CI) [2]	P (Q) [3]
Entire group; Global haplotype association *p*-value: 0.077										
H1	A	T	G	A	C	G	0.5215	0.4644	1.00	—
H2	A	C	G	A	T	G	0.1457	0.1878	**1.46 (1.14–1.87)**	**0.003 (0.034)**
H3	G	T	A	A	T	A	0.1572	0.1755	**1.30 (1.02–1.66)**	**0.036** (0.28)
H4	A	T	G	A	T	G	0.0733	0.0762	1.25 (0.89–1.77)	0.20 (0.46)
H5	G	T	G	A	C	G	0.0290	0.0221	0.94 (0.54–1.63)	0.81 (0.93)
H6	G	T	A	A	C	A	0.0220	0.0202	1.05 (0.55–2.03)	0.88 (0.96)
H7	A	T	G	T	T	G	0.0181	0.0168	1.30 (0.66–2.56)	0.45 (0.74)
rare	*	*	*	*	*	*	0.0152	0.0063	1.18 (0.70–1.99)	0.54 (0.78)

Table 3. *Cont.*

Haplotype Number	rs4724800	rs7784465	rs10951982	rs10238136	rs836478	rs9374	T2D Patients: Without DR	T2D Patients: With DR	OR (95% CI) [2]	P (Q) [3]
							Haplotype Frequency [1]			
Males Global haplotype association *p*-value: **0.009**										
H1	A	T	G	A	C	G	0.5326	0.4438	1.00	—
H2	A	C	G	A	T	G	0.111	0.1839	**2.32 (1.46–3.67)**	**0.0004 (0.009)**
H3	G	T	A	A	T	A	0.1732	0.1689	1.14 (0.78–1.66)	0.50 (0.77)
H4	A	T	G	A	T	G	0.0800	0.1033	1.50 (0.90–2.51)	0.12 (0.39)
H5	G	T	G	A	C	G	0.0253	0.0213	1.03 (0.41–2.56)	0.95 (0.96)
H6	G	T	A	A	C	A	0.0138	0.0220	2.08 (0.63–6.90)	0.23 (0.48)
H7	A	T	G	T	T	G	0.0249	0.0240	1.13 (0.48–2.70)	0.78 (0.93)
H8	A	C	G	A	C	G	0.0241	0.0056	0.20 (0.04–1.03)	0.06 (0.29)
rare	*	*	*	*	*	*	0.0033	0.0030	2.19 (0.74–6.49)	0.16 (0.46)
Females Global haplotype association *p*-value: 0.22										
H1	A	T	G	A	C	G	0.4478	0.4745	1.00	—
H2	A	C	G	A	T	G	0.1659	0.1791	1.01 (0.74–1.38)	0.96 (0.96)
H3	G	T	A	A	T	A	0.1956	0.1582	0.75 (0.56–1.02)	0.07 (0.29)
H4	A	T	G	A	T	G	0.0765	0.0734	0.88 (0.56–1.39)	0.58 (0.78)
H5	G	T	G	A	C	G	0.0349	0.0203	0.56 (0.29–1.09)	0.09 (0.33)
H6	G	T	A	A	C	A	0.0244	0.0268	0.85 (0.37–1.92)	0.69 (0.88)
H7	A	T	G	T	T	G	0.0059	0.0180	0.57 (0.21–1.55)	0.27 (0.52)
H8	A	C	G	A	C	G	0.0195	0.0135	2.38 (0.63–9.02)	0.20 (0.46)
rare	*	*	*	*	*	*	0.0121	0.0063	1.49 (0.66–3.38)	0.34 (0.60)

[1] Rare haplotypes with frequency < 0.01 are not shown and indicated as "*". [2] Odds ratio with 95% confidence intervals adjusted for age, sex, and BMI (codominant genetic model). [3] *p*-value (FDR-adjusted *p*-value) adjusted for age, sex, and BMI. Bold is statistically significant *P*- and *Q*-values.

The frequency of the haplotypes *H2* rs4724800A-rs7784465C-rs10951982G-rs10238136A-rs836478T-rs9374G and *H3* rs4724800G-rs7784465T-rs10951982A-rs10238136A-rs836478T-rs9374A was significantly higher in the patients with DR. A sex-stratified analysis showed a much stronger association of the haplotype *H2* rs4724800A-rs7784465C-rs10951982G-rs10238136A-rs836478T-rs9374G with DR in diabetic males (OR 2.32, 95CI 1.46–3.67, $p = 0.0004$).

3.3. Polymorphisms of the RAC1 Gene and Diabetic Nephropathy

The minor allele rs836478-T was associated with DNF exclusively in males (OR 1.43, 95% CI 1.05–1.96, $p = 0.025$). The genotype frequencies for the studied SNPs in the diabetics with and without DNF are shown in Table 4.

Table 4. Genotype frequencies for the studied gene polymorphisms among T2D patients with and without diabetic nephropathy.

RAC1 SNP ID	Genotype	T2D Patients: Without DNF *n* (%)	T2D Patients: With DNF *n* (%)	*P* (Q) [1]	OR (95% CI) [2]
Entire group					
rs4724800 A>G	A/A	520 (59.5)	322 (58.4)	0.42 (0.74)	1.00
	A/G	315 (36)	197 (35.8)		1.04 (0.82–1.33)
	G/G	39 (4.5)	32 (5.8)		1.44 (0.84–2.47)
rs7784465 T>C	T/T	565 (65.8)	347 (64.6)	0.99 (0.99)	1.00
	T/C	261 (30.4)	169 (31.5)		1.00 (0.78–1.30)
	C/C	33 (3.8)	21 (3.9)		1.04 (0.56–1.91)
rs10951982 G>A	G/G	557 (63.7)	346 (63)	0.31 (0.74)	1.00
	G/A	284 (32.5)	173 (31.5)		0.99 (0.77–1.27)
	A/A	33 (3.8)	30 (5.5)		1.57 (0.88–2.81)
rs10238136 A>T	A/A	818 (94.1)	515 (95)	0.66 (0.85)	1.00
	A/T	50 (5.8)	26 (4.8)		0.81 (0.48–1.37)
	T/T	1 (0.1)	1 (0.2)		1.84 (0.11–30.29)
rs836478 C>T	C/C	262 (30.5)	162 (29.6)	0.60 (0.83)	1.00
	C/T	418 (48.7)	260 (47.5)		1.04 (0.79–1.36)
	T/T	179 (20.8)	125 (22.9)		1.18 (0.85–1.63)
rs9374 G>A	G/G	544 (63.5)	352 (64.2)	0.17 (0.74)	1.00
	G/A	286 (33.4)	169 (30.8)		0.94 (0.73–1.21)
	A/A	27 (3.1)	27 (4.9)		1.74 (0.93–3.25)

Table 4. *Cont.*

RAC1 SNP ID	Genotype	T2D Patients: Without DNF *n* (%)	T2D Patients: With DNF *n* (%)	*P* (*Q*) [1]	OR (95% CI) [2]
Males					
rs4724800 A>G	A/A	218 (58.8)	62 (61.4)	0.91 (0.96)	1.00
	A/G	130 (35)	33 (32.7)		0.90 (0.55–1.48)
	G/G	23 (6.2)	6 (5.9)		0.91 (0.34–2.43)
rs7784465 T>C	T/T	246 (68.5)	62 (63.3)	0.56 (0.83)	1.00
	T/C	103 (28.7)	34 (34.7)		1.32 (0.80–2.16)
	C/C	10 (2.8)	2 (2)		1.03 (0.21–5.01)
rs10951982 G>A	G/G	237 (63.4)	66 (66)	0.40 (0.74)	1.00
	G/A	118 (31.6)	27 (27)		0.78 (0.47–1.32)
	A/A	19 (5.1)	7 (7)		1.50 (0.58–3.90)
rs10238136 A>T	A/A	346 (94)	93 (93)	0.28 (0.74)	1.00
	A/T	22 (6)	6 (6)		1.15 (0.44–3.03)
	T/T	0 (0)	1 (1)		NA
rs836478 C>T	C/C	115 (31.2)	21 (21.2)	0.056 (0.74)	1.00
	C/T	179 (48.5)	50 (50.5)		1.70 (0.95–3.04)
	T/T	75 (20.3)	28 (28.3)		**2.16 (1.12–4.17)**
rs9374 G>A	G/G	233 (63)	64 (64.7)	0.29 (0.74)	1.00
	G/A	121 (32.7)	28 (28.3)		0.80 (0.47–1.33)
	A/A	16 (4.3)	7 (7.1)		1.81 (0.67–4.86)
Females					
rs4724800 A>G	A/A	302 (60)	260 (57.8)	0.22 (0.74)	1.00
	A/G	185 (36.8)	164 (36.4)		1.10 (0.83–1.46)
	G/G	16 (3.2)	26 (5.8)		1.80 (0.91–3.57)
rs7784465 T>C	T/T	319 (63.8)	285 (64.9)	0.82 (0.92)	1.00
	T/C	158 (31.6)	135 (30.8)		0.91 (0.68–1.23)
	C/C	23 (4.6)	19 (4.3)		1.02 (0.52–1.99)
rs10951982 G>A	G/G	320 (64)	280 (62.4)	0.45 (0.74)	1.00
	G/A	166 (33.2)	146 (32.5)		1.07 (0.80–1.44)
	A/A	14 (2.8)	23 (5.1)		1.57 (0.76–3.25)
rs10238136 A>T	A/A	472 (94.2)	422 (95.5)	0.32 (0.74)	1.00
	A/T	28 (5.6)	20 (4.5)		0.71 (0.38–1.31)
	T/T	1 (0.2)	0 (0)		NA
rs836478 C>T	C/C	147 (30)	141 (31.5)	0.77 (0.92)	1.00
	C/T	239 (48.8)	210 (46.9)		0.90 (0.65–1.23)
	T/T	104 (21.2)	97 (21.6)		0.97 (0.66–1.42)
rs9374 G>A	G/G	311 (63.9)	288 (64.1)	0.44 (0.74)	1.00
	G/A	165 (33.9)	141 (31.4)		0.99 (0.74–1.33)
	A/A	11 (2.3)	20 (4.5)		1.67 (0.75–3.73)

[1] *p*-value (FDR-adjusted *p*-value) adjusted for age, sex, and BMI. [2] Odds ratio with 95% confidence intervals adjusted for age, sex, and BMI (codominant genetic model). Bold is statistically significant *P*- and *Q*-values.

As can be seen from Table 4, the polymorphism rs836478 was associated with the risk of DNF in males in the codominant model. However, the rs836478-C/T-T/T genotypes of *RAC1* were found to be associated with an increased risk of diabetic nephropathy in male diabetics (OR 1.84, 95% CI 1.06–3.19, $p = 0.024$) in the dominant model. The other SNPs of the *RAC1* gene showed no significant associations with a DNF risk. A haplotype analysis (Supplementary Table S1) revealed that none of the *RAC1* haplotypes were associated with diabetic nephropathy.

3.4. *RAC1* Gene Polymorphisms and the Risk of Diabetic Neuropathy

The frequencies of the minor alleles rs7784465-C (OR 1.80, 95% CI 1.17–2.75, $p = 0.007$) and rs836478-T (OR 1.35, 95% CI 1.02–1.80, $p = 0.037$) were significantly higher in the patients with DN compared to the patients without DN. The allele rs7784465-C was also associated with DN in females (OR 2.02, 95% CI 1.08–3.76, $p = 0.028$). The genotype frequencies of the *RAC1* gene polymorphisms among the T2D patients with and without diabetic neuropathy are given in Table 5.

Table 5. Genotype frequencies for the studied gene polymorphisms among T2D patients with and without diabetic neuropathy.

RAC1 SNP ID	Genotype	T2D Patients Without DN *n* (%)	With DN *n* (%)	*P* (*Q*) [1]	OR (95% CI) [2]
Entire group					
rs4724800 A>G	A/A	69 (65.1)	766 (59.1)	0.62 (0.73)	1.00
	A/G	33 (31.1)	466 (35.9)		1.20 (0.76–1.87)
	G/G	4 (3.8)	65 (5)		1.44 (0.49–4.26)
rs7784465 T>C	T/T	83 (79)	817 (64.3)	**0.008** (0.13)	1.00
	T/C	19 (18.1)	403 (31.7)		**2.16 (1.27–3.67)**
	C/C	3 (2.9)	50 (3.9)		1.99 (0.57–6.96)
rs10951982 G>A	G/G	74 (69.2)	821 (63.4)	0.49 (0.73)	1.00
	G/A	27 (25.2)	418 (32.3)		1.29 (0.80–2.07)
	A/A	6 (5.6)	56 (4.3)		0.83 (0.33–2.11)
rs10238136 A>T	A/A	93 (91.2)	1219 (94.7)	0.29 (0.54)	1.00
	A/T	9 (8.8)	66 (5.1)		0.53 (0.24–1.14)
	T/T	0 (0)	2 (0.2)		NA
rs836478 C>T	C/C	40 (37.4)	380 (29.7)	0.097 (0.44)	1.00
	C/T	51 (47.7)	616 (48.2)		1.36 (0.86–2.15)
	T/T	16 (14.9)	282 (22.1)		1.94 (1.04–3.64)
rs9374 G>A	G/G	75 (69.4)	813 (63.7)	0.65 (0.73)	1.00
	G/A	29 (26.9)	415 (32.5)		1.24 (0.78–1.97)
	A/A	4 (3.7)	48 (3.8)		1.15 (0.38–3.47)
Males					
rs4724800 A>G	A/A	39 (68.4)	235 (59.6)	0.18 (0.46)	1.00
	A/G	17 (29.8)	133 (33.8)		1.29 (0.68–2.45)
	G/G	1 (1.8)	26 (6.6)		4.76 (0.58–38.95)
rs7784465 T>C	T/T	42 (76.4)	254 (66.5)	0.33 (0.54)	1.00
	T/C	12 (21.8)	118 (30.9)		1.61 (0.79–3.29)
	C/C	1 (1.8)	10 (2.6)		2.20 (0.26–19.02)
rs10951982 G>A	G/G	40 (70.2)	256 (64.5)	0.57 (0.73)	1.00
	G/A	15 (26.3)	118 (29.7)		1.17 (0.60–2.28)
	A/A	2 (3.5)	23 (5.8)		2.12 (0.44–10.23)
rs10238136 A>T	A/A	51 (92.7)	368 (93.9)	0.93 (0.93)	1.00
	A/T	4 (7.3)	23 (5.9)		0.87 (0.27–2.84)
	T/T	0 (0)	1 (0.3)		NA
rs836478 C>T	C/C	21 (36.2)	111 (28.5)	0.095 (0.44)	1.00
	C/T	30 (51.7)	189 (48.5)		1.39 (0.72–2.66)
	T/T	7 (12.1)	90 (23.1)		2.74 (1.05–7.15)
rs9374 G>A	G/G	40 (69)	250 (63.9)	0.32 (0.54)	1.00
	G/A	17 (29.3)	121 (30.9)		1.06 (0.56–2.02)
	A/A	1 (1.7)	20 (5.1)		3.99 (0.47–33.53)
Females					
rs4724800 A>G	A/A	30 (61.2)	531 (58.8)	0.69 (0.73)	1.00
	A/G	16 (32.6)	333 (36.9)		1.12 (0.59–2.11)
	G/G	3 (6.1)	39 (4.3)		0.62 (0.18–2.17)
rs7784465 T>C	T/T	41 (82)	563 (63.4)	**0.014** (0.13)	1.00
	T/C	7 (14)	285 (32.1)		**3.01 (1.31–6.91)**
	C/C	2 (4)	40 (4.5)		1.88 (0.41–8.72)
rs10951982 G>A	G/G	34 (68)	565 (62.9)	0.14 (0.46)	1.00
	G/A	12 (24)	300 (33.4)		1.44 (0.72–2.85)
	A/A	4 (8)	33 (3.7)		0.39 (0.13–1.20)
rs10238136 A>T	A/A	42 (89.4)	851 (95.1)	0.16 (0.46)	1.00
	A/T	5 (10.6)	43 (4.8)		0.34 (0.12–0.93)
	T/T	0 (0)	1 (0.1)		NA
rs836478 C>T	C/C	19 (38.8)	269 (30.3)	0.55 (0.73)	1.00
	C/T	21 (42.9)	427 (48.1)		1.38 (0.72–2.66)
	T/T	9 (18.4)	192 (21.6)		1.45 (0.63–3.34)
rs9374 G>A	G/G	35 (70)	563 (63.6)	0.23 (0.52)	1.00
	G/A	12 (24)	294 (33.2)		1.48 (0.75–2.93)
	A/A	3 (6)	28 (3.2)		0.46 (0.13–1.64)

[1] *p*-value (FDR-adjusted *p*-value) adjusted for age, sex, and BMI. [2] Odds ratio with 95% confidence intervals adjusted for age, sex, and BMI (codominant genetic model). Bold is statistically significant *P*- and *Q*-values.

The genotype rs7784465-T/C of *RAC1* was associated with an increased risk of DN in the entire group of T2D patients and diabetic females. As can be seen from Table 6, the haplotype *H2* rs4724800A-rs7784465C-rs10951982G-rs10238136A-rs836478T-rs9374G and the minor alleles rs7784465-C and rs836478-T were associated with an increased risk of DN in both diabetic males and females. Interestingly, the haplotype *H5* rs4724800G-rs7784465T-rs10951982G-rs10238136A-rs836478C-rs9374G showed an association with an increased risk of DN only in males. Meanwhile, the haplotype *H7* rs4724800A-rs7784465T-rs10951982G-rs10238136T-rs836478T-rs9374G possessed a protective effect against the DN risk in diabetic females.

Table 6. Estimated common haplotype frequencies of *RAC1* gene in T2D patients with and without diabetic neuropathy.

Haplotype Number	SNPs						T2D Patients		OR (95% CI) [2]	P (Q) [3]
	rs4724800	rs7784465	rs10951982	rs10238136	rs836478	rs9374	Without DN	With DN		
							Haplotype Frequency [1]			
Entire group Global haplotype association *p*-value: **0.036**										
H1	A	T	G	A	C	G	0.5517	0.4750	1.00	—
H2	A	C	G	A	T	G	0.0999	0.1815	**2.22 (1.34–3.68)**	**0.0019 (0.02)**
H3	G	T	A	A	T	A	0.1608	0.1713	1.20 (0.78–1.82)	0.41 (0.72)
H4	A	T	G	A	T	G	0.0889	0.0744	1.11 (0.63–1.94)	0.72 (0.95)
H5	G	T	G	A	C	G	0.0178	0.0237	1.37 (0.45–4.15)	0.58 (0.81)
H6	G	T	A	A	C	A	0.0105	0.0220	2.53 (0.59–10.85)	0.21 (0.60)
H7	A	T	G	T	T	G	0.0344	0.0155	0.58 (0.23–1.42)	0.23 (0.60)
rare	*	*	*	*	*	*	0.0106	0.0085	0.95 (0.40–2.26)	0.90 (0.96)
Males Global haplotype association *p*-value: 0.19										
H1	A	T	G	A	C	G	0.5715	0.4628	1.00	—
H2	A	C	G	A	T	G	0.1015	0.1637	**2.32 (1.10–4.92)**	**0.028** (0.15)
H3	G	T	A	A	T	A	0.1541	0.1747	1.52 (0.83–2.77)	0.17 (0.60)
H4	A	T	G	A	T	G	0.0990	0.0941	1.33 (0.62–2.84)	0.47 (0.76)
H5	G	T	G	A	C	G	0.0000	0.0213	**2.41 (1.28–6.18)**	**<0.0001 (0.002)**
H6	G	T	A	A	C	A	0.0097	0.0202	2.49 (0.31–20.32)	0.39 (0.72)
H7	A	T	G	T	T	G	0.0247	0.0252	1.52 (0.39–5.98)	0.55 (0.81)
rare	*	*	*	*	*	*	0.0106	0.0020	1.23 (0.25–6.07)	0.80 (0.96)
Females Global haplotype association *p*-value: **0.047**										
H1	A	T	G	A	C	G	0.5290	0.4807	1.00	—
H2	A	C	G	A	T	G	0.0968	0.1892	**2.13 (1.05–4.30)**	**0.036** (0.15)
H3	G	T	A	A	T	A	0.1686	0.1702	0.97 (0.53–1.76)	0.91 (0.96)
H4	A	T	G	A	T	G	0.0759	0.0661	0.94 (0.40–2.21)	0.88 (0.96)
H5	G	T	G	A	C	G	0.0374	0.0230	0.58 (0.18–1.88)	0.36 (0.72)
H6	G	T	A	A	C	A	0.0114	0.0222	2.36 (0.30–18.53)	0.41 (0.72)
H7	A	T	G	T	T	G	0.0477	0.0114	**0.20 (0.06–0.66)**	**0.009 (0.05)**
rare	*	*	*	*	*	*	0.0000	0.0069	1.01 (0.29–3.55)	0.99 (0.99)

[1] Rare haplotypes with frequency < 0.01 are not shown and indicated as "*". [2] Odds ratio with 95% confidence intervals adjusted for age, sex, and BMI (codominant genetic model). [3] *p*-value (FDR-adjusted *p*-value) adjusted for age, sex, and BMI. Bold is statistically significant *P*- and *Q*-values.

3.5. The Link between RAC1 Gene Polymorphisms to Diabetic Angiopathy of the Lower Extremities and Diabetic Foot Syndrome

The minor allele rs10238136-T was found to be associated with diabetic angiopathy of the lower extremities in females (OR 3.47, 95%CI 1.42–8.46, $p = 0.004$). The genotype frequencies for the *RAC1* gene polymorphisms among the T2D patients with and without diabetic angiopathy of the lower extremities are given in Table 7.

Table 7. Genotype frequencies for the studied *RAC1* gene polymorphisms among T2D patients with and without diabetic angiopathy of lower extremities.

RAC1 SNP ID	Genotype	T2D Patients Without DA n (%)	T2D Patients With DA n (%)	*P* (*Q*) [1]	OR (95% CI) [2]
		Entire group			
rs4724800 A>G	A/A A/G G/G	293 (59.4) 173 (35.1) 27 (5.5)	552 (57.4) 365 (37.9) 45 (4.7)	0.54 (0.94)	1.00 1.13 (0.89–1.43) 0.93 (0.55–1.56)
rs7784465 T>C	T/T T/C C/C	312 (65) 142 (29.6) 26 (5.4)	587 (62.7) 316 (33.8) 33 (3.5)	0.08 (0.36)	1.00 1.20 (0.93–1.54) 0.65 (0.37–1.13)
rs10951982 G>A	G/G G/A A/A	313 (63.2) 161 (32.5) 21 (4.2)	596 (62.3) 321 (33.5) 40 (4.2)	0.94 (0.94)	1.00 1.03 (0.81–1.31) 1.09 (0.62–1.94)
rs10238136 A>T	A/A A/T T/T	472 (96.5) 16 (3.3) 1 (0.2)	887 (93.8) 58 (6.1) 1 (0.1)	**0.02** (0.18)	1.00 **2.16 (1.20–3.87)** 0.45 (0.03–7.19)
rs836478 C>T	C/C C/T T/T	149 (30.6) 243 (49.9) 95 (19.5)	271 (28.6) 459 (48.4) 218 (23)	0.20 (0.60)	1.00 1.03 (0.79–1.34) 1.31 (0.95–1.81)
rs9374 G>A	G/G G/A A/A	311 (63.5) 159 (32.5) 20 (4.1)	592 (62.6) 322 (34) 32 (3.4)	0.88 (0.94)	1.00 1.05 (0.82–1.34) 0.93 (0.51–1.70)
		Males			
rs4724800 A>G	A/A A/G G/G	123 (60) 72 (35.1) 10 (4.9)	157 (57.7) 102 (37.5) 13 (4.8)	0.87 (0.94)	1.00 1.09 (0.74–1.62) 1.17 (0.47–2.93)
rs7784465 T>C	T/T T/C C/C	131 (65.5) 57 (28.5) 12 (6)	160 (60.1) 104 (39.1) 2 (0.8)	**0.031** (0.19)	1.00 **1.56 (1.04–2.33)** 0.16 (0.03–1.02)
rs10951982 G>A	G/G G/A A/A	130 (62.8) 68 (32.9) 9 (4.3)	171 (63.6) 86 (32) 12 (4.5)	0.91 (0.94)	1.00 0.94 (0.63–1.41) 1.15 (0.44–3.02)
rs10238136 A>T	A/A A/T T/T	192 (94.1) 11 (5.4) 1 (0.5)	249 (94) 16 (6) 0 (0)	0.27 (0.69)	1.00 1.13 (0.50–2.57) NA
rs836478 C>T	C/C C/T T/T	56 (27.4) 104 (51) 44 (21.6)	73 (27) 136 (50.4) 61 (22.6)	0.94 (0.94)	1.00 0.99 (0.64–1.55) 1.08 (0.63–1.86)
rs9374 G>A	G/G G/A A/A	130 (63.1) 68 (33) 8 (3.9)	172 (63.9) 86 (32) 11 (4.1)	0.91 (0.94)	1.00 0.94 (0.63–1.41) 1.17 (0.42–3.24)
		Females			
rs4724800 A>G	A/A A/G G/G	170 (59) 101 (35.1) 17 (5.9)	395 (57.2) 263 (38.1) 32 (4.6)	0.48 (0.94)	1.00 1.16 (0.86–1.56) 0.83 (0.45–1.56)
rs7784465 T>C	T/T T/C C/C	181 (64.6) 85 (30.4) 14 (5)	427 (63.7) 212 (31.6) 31 (4.6)	0.92 (0.94)	1.00 1.05 (0.77–1.44) 0.93 (0.48–1.83)
rs10951982 G>A	G/G G/A A/A	183 (63.5) 93 (32.3) 12 (4.2)	425 (61.8) 235 (34.2) 28 (4.1)	0.86 (0.94)	1.00 1.09 (0.80–1.47) 1.08 (0.53–2.19)
rs10238136 A>T	A/A A/T T/T	280 (98.2) 5 (1.8) 0 (0)	638 (93.7) 42 (6.2) 1 (0.2)	**0.0019 (0.034)**	1.00 **4.14 (1.60–10.69)** NA
rs836478 C>T	C/C C/T T/T	93 (32.9) 139 (49.1) 51 (18)	198 (29.2) 323 (47.6) 157 (23.2)	0.12 (0.43)	1.00 1.04 (0.75–1.44) 1.48 (0.98–2.23)
rs9374 G>A	G/G G/A A/A	181 (63.7) 91 (32) 12 (4.2)	420 (62) 236 (34.9) 21 (3.1)	0.64 (0.94)	1.00 1.12 (0.83–1.53) 0.83 (0.40–1.76)

[1] *p*-value (FDR-adjusted *p*-value) adjusted for age, sex, and BMI. [2] Odds ratio with 95% confidence intervals adjusted for age, sex, and BMI (codominant genetic model). Bold is statistically significant *P*- and *Q*-values.

The genotype rs10238136-A/T was associated with an increased risk of DA in the entire group and in diabetic females, whereas the genotype rs7784465-T/C was associated with DA only in males. Meanwhile, the haplotype *H7* rs4724800A-rs7784465T-rs10951982G-rs10238136T-rs836478T-rs9374G (Table 8) showed an association with an increased risk of DA in females.

Table 8. Estimated common haplotype frequencies of *RAC1* gene in T2D patients with and without diabetic angiopathy of lower extremities.

Haplotype Number	SNPs						T2D Patients		OR (95% CI) [2]	P (Q) [3]
	rs4724800	rs7784465	rs10951982	rs10238136	rs836478	rs9374	Without DA	With DA		
							Haplotype Frequency [1]			
Entire group Global haplotype association *p*-value: 0.53										
H1	A	T	G	A	C	G	0.4869	0.4595	1.00	—
H2	A	C	G	A	T	G	0.1665	0.1831	1.13 (0.89–1.42)	0.31 (0.67)
H3	G	T	A	A	T	A	0.1601	0.1776	1.20 (0.95–1.52)	0.12 (0.67)
H4	A	T	G	A	T	G	0.0757	0.0756	1.00 (0.72–1.38)	0.99 (0.99)
H5	G	T	G	A	C	G	0.0241	0.0238	1.12 (0.63–1.98)	0.70 (0.86)
H6	G	T	A	A	C	A	0.0212	0.0210	0.78 (0.42–1.43)	0.41 (0.67)
H7	A	T	G	T	T	G	0.0123	0.0181	1.78 (0.84–3.76)	0.13 (0.67)
H8	A	C	G	A	C	G	0.0146	0.0115	0.74 (0.33–1.66)	0.46 (0.67)
rare	*	*	*	*	*	*	0.0099	0.0026	0.93 (0.55–1.59)	0.79 (0.86)
Males Global haplotype association *p*-value: 0.83										
H1	A	T	G	A	C	G	0.4889	0.4569	1.00	—
H2	A	C	G	A	T	G	0.1775	0.1808	1.05 (0.71–1.53)	0.82 (0.86)
H3	G	T	A	A	T	A	0.1736	0.1908	1.16 (0.80–1.70)	0.44 (0.67)
H4	A	T	G	A	T	G	0.0634	0.0810	1.28 (0.75–2.20)	0.37 (0.67)
H5	G	T	G	A	C	G	0.0202	0.0260	1.50 (0.58–3.87)	0.40 (0.67)
H6	A	T	G	T	T	G	0.0209	0.0158	0.67 (0.24–1.82)	0.43 (0.67)
rare	*	*	*	*	*	*	0.0058	0.0121	0.88 (0.46–1.68)	0.70 (0.86)
Females Global haplotype association *p*-value: 0.078										
H1	A	T	G	A	C	G	0.4904	0.4615	1.00	—
H2	A	C	G	A	T	G	0.1576	0.1838	1.15 (0.86–1.53)	0.36 (0.67)
H3	G	T	A	A	T	A	0.1473	0.1726	1.27 (0.94–1.72)	0.12 (0.67)
H4	A	T	G	A	T	G	0.0834	0.0731	0.83 (0.55–1.25)	0.38 (0.67)
H5	G	T	G	A	C	G	0.0285	0.0220	0.83 (0.42–1.63)	0.58 (0.80)
H6	G	T	A	A	C	A	0.0301	0.0251	0.63 (0.31–1.27)	0.2 (0.67)
H7	A	T	G	T	T	G	0.0057	0.0186	**4.63 (1.27–16.84)**	**0.02** (0.44)
H8	A	C	G	A	C	G	0.0186	0.0115	0.65 (0.24–1.71)	0.38 (0.67)
rare	*	*	*	*	*	*	0.0193	0.0034	1.11 (0.56–2.21)	0.76 (0.86)

[1] Rare haplotypes with frequency < 0.01 are not shown. [2] Odds ratio with 95% confidence intervals adjusted for age, sex, and BMI (codominant genetic model). [3] *p*-value (FDR-adjusted *p*-value) adjusted for age, sex, and BMI. Bold is statistically significant *P*- and *Q*-values.

As can be seen from Supplementary Table S2, none of the studied SNPs of the *RAC1* gene showed an association with the risk of diabetic foot syndrome. However, the minor allele rs10238136-T (OR 3.67, 95%CI 1.48–9.10, $p = 0.016$) and haplotype *H6* rs4724800A-rs7784465T-rs10951982G-rs10238136T-rs836478T-rs9374G (Table 9) were associated with diabetic foot syndrome in males.

Table 9. Estimated common haplotype frequencies of *RAC1* gene in T2D patients with and without diabetic foot syndrome.

Haplotype Number	SNPs						T2D Patients		OR (95% CI) [2]	*P* (*Q*) [3]
	rs4724800	rs7784465	rs10951982	rs10238136	rs836478	rs9374	Without DFS	With DFS		
							Haplotype Frequency [1]			
Entire group Global haplotype association *p*-value: 0.12										
H1	A	T	G	A	C	G	0.4642	0.4798	1.00	—
H2	A	C	G	A	T	G	0.1754	0.2227	1.23 (0.85–1.78)	0.26 (0.90)
H3	G	T	A	A	T	A	0.1739	0.1467	0.82 (0.54–1.25)	0.36 (0.90)
H4	A	T	G	A	T	G	0.0781	0.0477	0.56 (0.28–1.12)	0.10 (0.55)
H5	G	T	G	A	C	G	0.0239	0.0188	0.70 (0.24–2.08)	0.52 (0.94)
H6	G	T	A	A	C	A	0.0205	0.0286	1.25 (0.47–3.35)	0.65 (0.94)
H7	A	T	G	T	T	G	0.0153	0.0341	2.07 (0.91–4.70)	0.083 (0.55)
H8	A	C	G	A	C	G	0.0141	NA	NA	NA
rare	*	*	*	*	*	*	0.0055	0.0022	0.67 (0.23–1.91)	0.45 (0.90)
Males Global haplotype association *p*-value: 0.22										
H1	A	T	G	A	C	G	0.4677	0.4379	1.00	—
H2	A	C	G	A	T	G	0.1819	0.1999	1.19 (0.58–2.43)	0.64 (0.94)
H3	G	T	A	A	T	A	0.1845	0.1585	1.01 (0.48–2.14)	0.98 (1.0)
H4	A	T	G	A	T	G	0.0769	0.0750	1.01 (0.36–2.83)	0.98 (1.0)
H5	G	T	G	A	C	G	0.0252	NA	NA	NA
H6	A	T	G	T	T	G	0.0162	0.0632	**4.07 (1.20–13.82)**	**0.025** (0.55)
rare	*	*	*	*	*	*	0.0083	0.0000	1.56 (0.52–4.67)	0.42 (0.90)
Females Global haplotype association *p*-value: 0.099										
H1	A	T	G	A	C	G	0.4640	0.4986	1.00	—
H2	A	C	G	A	T	G	0.1725	0.2325	1.24 (0.81–1.90)	0.33 (0.90)
H3	G	T	A	A	T	A	0.1688	0.1410	0.80 (0.48–1.35)	0.40 (0.90)
H4	A	T	G	A	T	G	0.0781	0.0360	0.40 (0.16–1.03)	0.06 (0.55)
H5	G	T	G	A	C	G	0.0235	0.0274	1.08 (0.37–3.15)	0.89 (1.0)
H6	G	T	A	A	C	A	0.0261	0.0371	1.24 (0.44–3.51)	0.68 (0.94)
H7	A	T	G	T	T	G	0.0149	0.0202	1.36 (0.41–4.54)	0.61 (0.94)
H8	A	C	G	A	C	G	0.0159	NA	NA	NA
rare	*	*	*	*	*	*	0.0078	0.0000	0.22 (0.03–1.63)	0.14 (0.62)

[1] Rare haplotypes with frequency < 0.01 are not shown and indicated as "*". [2] Odds ratio with 95% confidence intervals adjusted for age, sex, and BMI (codominant genetic model). [3] *p*-value (FDR-adjusted *p*-value) adjusted for age, sex, and BMI. Bold is statistically significant *P*- and *Q*-values.

3.6. The Link between RAC1 Gene Haplotypes and Plasma Parameters of Redox Homeostasis

An analysis of the relationship between the genetic and biochemical parameters of redox homeostasis (Supplementary Table S3) revealed an association of the haplotype rs4724800A-rs7784465T-rs10951982G-rs10238136A-rs836478T-rs9374G with increased levels of ROS in the plasma of diabetics with DR (Diff = 1.02, 95% CI 0.18–1.85, $p = 0.017$), DNF (Diff = 1.14, 95% CI 0.26–2.02, $p = 0.011$) and DN (Diff = 0.90, 95% CI 0.25–1.55, $p = 0.0069$). Moreover, DNF patients carrying the same *RAC1* haplotype had a lower concentration of total plasma glutathione (Diff = −1.72, 95% CI −3.01–−0.44, $p = 0.0095$) compared with the carriers of the reference haplotype rs4724800A-rs7784465T-rs10951982G-rs10238136A-rs836478C-rs9374G.

The haplotype rs4724800A-rs7784465C-rs10951982G-rs10238136A-rs836478C-rs9374G was associated with higher ROS levels in patients with DNF (Diff = 6.82, 95% CI 4.90–8.73, $p < 0.0001$), DN (Diff = 5.73, 95% CI 4.44–7.01, $p < 0.0001$), and DA (Diff = 7.23, 95% CI 5.83–8.62, $p < 0.0001$). In patients with DFS, the haplotype rs4724800G-rs7784465C-rs10951982A-rs10238136A-rs836478T-rs9374A was associated with increased ROS (Diff = 4.10, 95% CI 2.52–5.68, $p < 0.0001$), whereas the carriers of the haplotypes rs4724800A-rs7784465C-rs10951982G-rs10238136A-rs836478T-rs9374G (Diff = 1.09, 95% CI 0.29–1.90, $p = 0.012$) and rs4724800G-rs7784465T-rs10951982A-rs10238136A-rs836478T-rs9374A (Diff = 1.03, 95% CI 0.08–1.98, $p = 0.039$) had higher levels of total glutathione in their blood plasma (Supplementary Table S3).

4. Discussion

4.1. Summary of the Study Findings

The present study found, for the first time, that the polymorphisms of the gene encoding Rac family small GTPase 1 (*RAC1*) in type 2 diabetes are associated with complications such as diabetic retinopathy, neuropathy, and angiopathy of the lower extremities. However, the observed associations were sex-specific. In particular, the genotype rs7784465-T/C was associated with an increased risk of retinopathy and angiopathy of the lower extremities in males, as well as diabetic neuropathy in females. Furthermore, the polymorphism rs836478 of *RAC1* was linked to diabetic retinopathy and nephropathy in males, whereas the polymorphism rs10238136 was linked to diabetic angiopathy in females. Figure 1 depicts the structure of the *RAC1* gene, the genomic position of the SNPs, and the haplotype structure of the gene, as well as summarizing the overall research findings. The *RAC1* haplotypes were found to be associated with DR in males and with DN in females. Furthermore, the *RAC1* haplotype rs4724800A-rs7784465C-rs10951982G-rs10238136A-rs836478T-rs9374G showed an association with DR in males and DN regardless of sex. In addition, the haplotype rs4724800A-rs7784465T-rs10951982G-rs10238136T-rs836478T-rs9374G was associated with a 4-fold risk of DA in females and DFS in males. The haplotype rs4724800A-rs7784465T-rs10951982G-rs10238136A-rs836478T-rs9374G showed an association with the increased plasma levels of ROS in diabetics with DR, DNF, and DN. The patients with DNF who carried the above haplotype had lower concentrations of total plasma glutathione. Moreover, the haplotype rs4724800A-rs7784465C-rs10951982G-rs10238136A-rs836478C-rs9374G was associated with higher ROS levels in patients with DNF, DN, and DA. The haplotype rs4724800G-rs7784465C-rs10951982A-rs10238136A-rs836478T-rs9374A was correlated with the increased ROS in patients with DFS, whereas the haplotypes rs4724800A-rs7784465C-rs10951982G-rs10238136A-rs836478T-rs9374G and rs4724800G-rs7784465T-rs10951982A-rs10238136A-rs836478T-rs9374A were correlated with the increased levels of total glutathione in the plasma. A functional annotation of the studied SNPs [20] showed that the minor alleles rs7784465-C, rs10951982-A, rs10238136-T, rs836478-T, and rs9374-A were associated with the increased expression of the *RAC1* gene in various tissues and might be binding sites for transcription factors (TF). For instance, an analysis of the TF-binding affinity of the rs836478 polymorphism (which was associated with DNF) with the atSNP tool [26] (http://atsnp.biostat.wisc.edu/search, accessed on 2 November 2020) has shown that the minor allele rs836478-T was predicted to create binding sites for 34 TFs, including FOXC1, FOXD1, PBX1, GATA3, and POU3F3, which are enriched with GO terms that are related to the development of the nephron epithelium and renal tubules, as assessed by the STRING database [27] (https://string-db.org/, accessed on 14 December 2022).

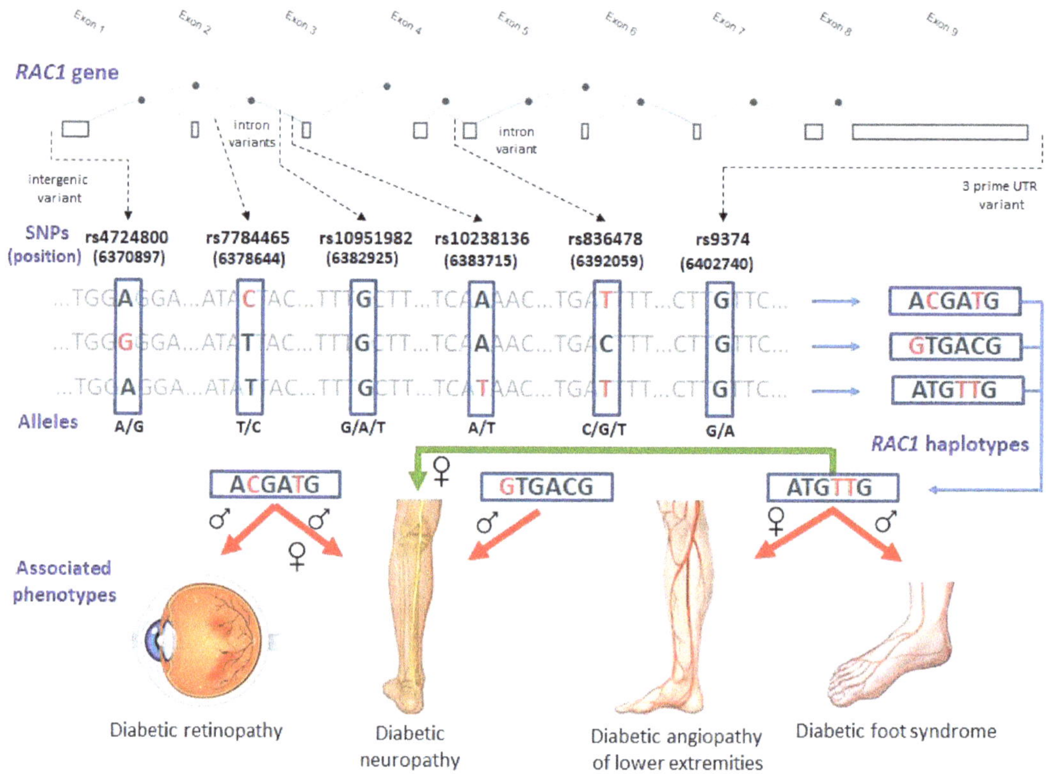

Figure 1. The exon–intron organization of the *RAC1* gene, SNP position, haplotype structure, and a summary of the observed associations.

Although many hypotheses have been proposed to explain the molecular pathways underlying diabetic complications, it is widely accepted that glutathione deficiency, the increased production of reactive oxygen species, and its resulting oxidative stress are the major pathological processes responsible for the development of diabetic complications [28–32].

4.2. Diabetic Retinopathy

Diabetic retinopathy is one of the most common complications of diabetes mellitus and is a major global contributor to vision loss and blindness [33,34]. According to a meta-analysis of large, population-based studies, the prevalence and progression of diabetic retinopathy have been linked to the serum levels of HbA1c, total cholesterol, and blood pressure, but only in about 10% of patients with type 2 diabetes [35], suggesting that other factors exist that explain the development of diabetic retinopathy in the majority of diabetics. Numerous studies [18,29,31,36] have shown that oxidative stress plays a key role in the onset of diabetic retinopathy. RAC1 is required for NADPH oxidase 2, an enzyme that generates reactive oxygen species. The transcriptional activity of the *RAC1* gene may be regulated through epigenetic mechanisms. In particular, Kowluru and co-workers observed that the histone mark H3K9me3 at the *Rac1* promoter assists with active DNA methylation-hydroxymethylation reactions, activating *Rac1* gene transcription in diabetic mice [19]. Cells that were exposed to high glucose concentrations were found to exhibit increased signaling in the chain Rac1–Nox2–ROS, increased levels of *Rac1* transcripts, and increased 5-hydroxymethylcytosine levels at the gene promoter [37]. ROS overproduction has been shown to speed up the loss of capillary cells and to cause retinal neurodegeneration through mitochondrial damage, whereas the inhibition of ROS production was found to inhibit caspase-3-mediated neuronal apoptosis and to prevent vision loss [38,39].

4.3. Diabetic Nephropathy

Diabetic nephropathy is a clinical syndrome that is characterized by persistent albuminuria and a progressive decline in renal function [40]. DNF is thought to be the most common cause of end-stage renal disease, affecting 20% to 50% of people with diabetes. The mechanisms of DNF are very complex, and despite decades of intensive research, the pathogenesis of this complication in type 2 diabetes is still not fully understood [41,42]. Numerous pathways, processes, molecules, and conditions, such as oxidative stress, the renin-angiotensin-aldosterone system, mitogen-activated protein kinases, the formation of advanced glycosylation end products (AGE), connective tissue growth factor, transforming growth factor beta-1 (TGF-β), and inflammatory cytokines, are known to contribute to the onset and progression of DNF [43–45]. The pathways and mediators that are involved in kidney damage in type 2 diabetes share a lot of overlaps. For instance, it has been discovered that oxidative stress damages the kidneys through the activation of the renin-angiotensin-aldosterone system, whereas angiotensin-II itself is capable of causing renal injury through oxidative stress [42]. Another example is NADPH oxidase stimulating the production of TGF-β, which stimulates the production of ROS via NADPH oxidase activation [41]. The experimental observation that the inhibition of oxidative stress improved a renal feature associated with streptozotocin-induced DNF has highlighted the role of oxidative stress in the induction and progression of DNF [46,47]. Meanwhile, oxidative stress can damage cells indirectly by activating other pathological pathways which damage the renal cells through unknown mechanisms [48]. Metabolic and hemodynamic alterations in the kidneys are also linked to oxidative stress, and both have additive detrimental effects on the organ [49].

The direct and indirect mechanisms by which oxidative stress causes kidney damage in diabetes have been proposed. ROS were found to cause direct damage to podocytes, mesangial cells, and endothelial cells, leading to proteinuria and tubule-interstitial fibrosis [50]. The mechanism of this damage was argued to be that the glomerulus, the filtering unit of the kidney, is more sensitive to oxidative injury than the other parts of the nephron [51]. Hyperglycemia is known to induce ROS production and oxidative damage to DNA, lipids, and proteins [52]. Chronic hyperglycemia can cause oxidative stress by increasing angiotensin-II levels, activating protein kinases, and increasing TGF-β expression [53]. For instance, increased angiotensin-II levels induce ROS production in the kidneys through the activation of NADPH oxidase [54]. It is observed that the ROS-associated activation of TGF-β causes the excessive remodeling of the extracellular matrix in the mesangium and promotes fibrotic processes in the kidneys [55]. As mentioned above, the increased production of ROS via NADPH oxidase in diabetes is attributed to the activation of the NF-κB pathway, which also promotes the transcriptional activation of the genes encoding inflammatory cytokines, thereby contributing to kidney injury and leading to renal fibrosis and a decline in renal function [56–58]. The activation of the α and β isoforms of protein kinases C is also known to induce oxidative damage to the kidneys through the increased production of NADPH-dependent superoxide anion radicals [59]. There are many other redox-sensitive signal transduction pathways, such as c-Jun N-terminal kinase (JNK), p38 MAP kinase, and the transcription factor activator protein 1 (AP-1), determining a vicious cycle between inflammation and oxidative stress [60,61].

We have established, for the first time, an association between the minor allele rs836478-T and an increased risk of diabetic nephropathy. According to the GTEx portal (https://gtexportal.org, accessed on 24 February 2023), the *RAC1* gene is expressed at a relatively high level in the kidneys, suggesting an important role of the Rac family small GTPase 1 in this organ. There have been no studies on humans or animals that have investigated the expression level of the *RAC1* gene in diabetic nephropathy, but there are studies that have investigated other NOX enzymes. In particular, an increased NOX-4 expression in renal cells was discovered in streptozotocin-induced diabetic rats [62], and subsequent studies have argued that up-regulated NOX-4 is the primary source of the increased ROS production in the kidneys that contributes to renal fibrosis and DNF [63]. Both the deletion and the inhibition of the NOX4 and NOX1 genes have been shown to be renoprotective [64]. Finally, Ying and co-workers have recently observed that the binding of RAC1 to the pyrin domain containing 3 (NLRP3) activates the NLRP3 inflammasome in the kidney and accelerates the pathological processes underlying diabetic nephropathy [65]. The above studies clearly demonstrate the importance of RAC1-mediated oxidative stress for the development of diabetic nephropathy.

4.4. Diabetic Angiopathy of Lower Extremities

Diabetic angiopathy of the lower extremities is a change in the structure of the vessels of the legs in patients with diabetes mellitus, in the form of a decrease in the elasticity of the vascular wall and its thickening, leading to the narrowing of the lumen or the complete obliteration of the arteries. Increased oxidative stress is implicated in the pathogenesis of the various vascular complications of diabetes, including in diabetic angiopathy of the lower extremities [66–68]. It is well-known that abnormal endothelial-dependent vasodilation in diabetic patients is at least partially attributed to the reactive oxygen species that are primarily generated by up-regulated NOXs and downregulated endothelial nitric oxide synthase [69,70]. The increase in ROS levels and the decrease in nitric oxide are known to cause irreversible damage to the vascular endothelial cells through apoptosis [68]. The increased expression of NOX subunits, such as p22phox, p47phox, and p67phox, and the associated increased production of vascular superoxide anion radicals have been identified in diabetic subjects [71].

4.5. Diabetic Neuropathy

Diabetic neuropathy is a unique neurodegenerative disorder of the peripheral nervous system that preferentially targets sensory axons, autonomic axons, and later, to a lesser extent, motor axons [72]. The peripheral neurons that supply the feet are the longest cells in the body and require a properly functioning vascular supply, mitochondria, and glucose and lipid metabolism [73]. The duration of the diabetes and the plasma levels of the HBA1c are considered to be major predictors of diabetic neuropathy [74]. We revealed an association of the genotype rs7784465-T/C of the *RAC1* gene with an increased risk of diabetic neuropathy in females. Female sex was found to be a risk factor for painful diabetic neuropathy, which is consistent with our findings [75]. The overproduction of superoxide anions has even been implicated in diabetic microvascular complications [76]. ROS production inhibits the GAPDH enzyme (glyceraldehyde-3-phosphate dehydrogenase) activity, causing upstream glycolytic metabolites to be diverted into the molecular pathways of glucose overutilization [77]. It is known that ROS production overwhelms the endogenous antioxidant defense in diabetic peripheral neuropathy, impairing the neural blood flow, nerve conduction, neurotrophic support, and neuronal mitochondrial function [78,79]. Hyperglycemia-induced oxidative and/or nitrosative stress causes DNA damage and the subsequent hyperactivation of poly(ADP-ribose) polymerases (PARP), which are the enzymes involved in DNA repair, cellular proliferation, and programmed cell death [80]. Overactivated PARPs consume NAD+, slowing glycolysis and impairing ATP function, as well as inhibiting GAPDH. PARP activation also promotes the formation of excess amounts of the superoxide anions and peroxynitrites that are associated with endothelial dysfunction, decreased nerve blood flow, neuronal energy deficit, a loss of nerve fiber density, and nerve conduction slowing [81,82].

4.6. Diabetic Foot Syndrome

Diabetic foot syndrome is a long-term complication of type 2 diabetes that is caused by a combination of vascular and neurological deterioration [83]. Epidemiological studies have shown that neuropathy is responsible for about 50% of the cases of diabetic foot syndrome [84]. Our study revealed that the *RAC1* haplotype rs4724800A-rs7784465T-rs10951982G-rs10238136T-rs836478T-rs9374G was associated with a four-fold risk of DFS in males. The study of Rossboth S. and co-workers found a positive association of DFS with the male sex [85]. The pathogenesis of DFS has been linked to a variety of conditions, including oxidative stress, the malfunction of polyol and inositol metabolism, increased Na/K-ATPase activity, endoneural microvascular deficits and ischemia, defective axonal transport, and the non-enzymatic glycosylation of proteins in peripheral neurons [86,87].

The study has some limitations. Because the sample size of the patients with a specific diabetic complication was relatively small, the statistical power of the association analysis that was performed in the subgroups was decreased. A limited number of patients undergoing biochemical investigations of their redox homeostasis did not allow for the obtainment of more reliable estimates of the effects of the studied SNPs on these parameters in subgroups with particular diabetic complications. This limitation made it difficult to interpret the revealed associations between the *RAC1* haplotypes and the plasma levels of the ROS and total glutathione. Furthermore, there may be other unexplored confounding variables in the diabetics that contribute to the development of diabetic complications.

5. Conclusions

The present study demonstrated, for the first time, that the genetic variants in the *RAC1* gene represent novel susceptibility markers for diabetic retinopathy, nephropathy, angiopathy of the lower extremities, and neuropathy, with the potential to influence the risk of diabetic complications through perturbations in redox homeostasis. The sexual dimorphism of the associations between the *RAC1* gene polymorphisms and the risk of diabetic retinopathy, particularly in men, appears to be due to the male sex itself being a known risk factor for this complication [85,88]. The mechanisms underlying the sex-specific associations of these genetic polymorphisms with a susceptibility for common diseases are a hallmark of research and continue to pique the interest of scientists [89,90]. The associations of the *RAC1* gene haplotypes with the elevated concentrations of reactive oxygen species in patients with diabetic retinopathy, nephropathy, neuropathy, angiopathy, and diabetic foot syndrome may be intermediate damaging factors underlying the development of microvascular and nerve tissue diabetic complications. Because this is the first study to look into the role of the *RAC1* gene polymorphisms in diabetic complications, there are no comparable studies to compare our findings to. Further studies into other populations of the world are required to validate these associations between the polymorphisms of the *RAC1* gene and diabetic complications. However, our findings can already be applied to the development of new pharmacological agents that inhibit the RAC1 expression in specific tissues and thus reduce the ROS production.

Supplementary Materials: The following supporting information can be downloaded at: https://www.mdpi.com/article/10.3390/biomedicines11030981/s1, Table S1: Estimated common haplotype frequencies of *RAC1* gene in T2D patients with and without DNF; Table S2: Genotype frequencies for the studied *RAC1* gene polymorphisms among T2D patients with and without diabetic foot syndrome (DFS); Table S3: Associations of *RAC1* haplotypes with plasma redox homeostasis parameters.

Author Contributions: Conceptualization, A.P.; methodology, I.A., E.K. and A.P.; software, I.A. and A.P.; validation, A.P.; formal analysis, I.A. and A.P.; investigation, I.A., E.K. and A.P.; resources, I.A.; data curation, I.A., E.K. and A.P.; writing—original draft preparation, I.A. and A.P.; writing—review and editing, A.P. and I.A.; visualization, A.P. and I.A.; supervision, A.P.; project administration, A.P.; funding acquisition, I.A., E.K. and A.P. All authors have read and agreed to the published version of the manuscript.

Funding: This research was funded by the Russian Science Foundation under Grant no. 20-15-00227.

Institutional Review Board Statement: The study was conducted in accordance with the Declaration of Helsinki, and approved by the Regional Ethics Committee of Kursk State Medical University (protocol No.10, date: 12 December 2016).

Informed Consent Statement: Informed consent was obtained from all subjects involved in the study.

Data Availability Statement: Data supporting reported results are available upon request.

Acknowledgments: We thank all patients with type 2 diabetes and stuff of the Kursk Emergency Hospital.

Conflicts of Interest: The authors declare no conflict of interest.

References

1. Sun, H.; Saeedi, P.; Karuranga, S.; Pinkepank, M.; Ogurtsova, K.; Duncan, B.B.; Stein, C.; Basit, A.; Chan, J.C.; Mbanya, J.C.; et al. IDF Diabetes Atlas: Global, regional and country-level diabetes prevalence estimates for 2021 and projections for 2045. *Diabetes Res. Clin. Pract.* **2022**, *183*, 109119. [CrossRef] [PubMed]
2. Sinclair, A.; Saeedi, P.; Kaundal, A.; Karuranga, S.; Malanda, B.; Williams, R. Diabetes and global ageing among 65–99-year-old adults: Findings from the International Diabetes Federation Diabetes Atlas, 9th edition. *Diabetes Res. Clin. Pract.* **2020**, *162*, 108078. [CrossRef]
3. Azarova, I.; Polonikov, A.; Klyosova, E. Molecular Genetics of Abnormal Redox Homeostasis in Type 2 Diabetes Mellitus. *Int. J. Mol. Sci.* **2023**, *24*, 4738. [CrossRef] [PubMed]
4. Singh, A.; Kukreti, R.; Saso, L.; Kukreti, S. Mechanistic Insight into Oxidative Stress-Triggered Signaling Pathways and Type 2 Diabetes. *Molecules* **2022**, *27*, 950. [CrossRef]
5. Azarova, I.; Klyosova, E.; Polonikov, A. The Link between Type 2 Diabetes Mellitus and the Polymorphisms of Glutathione-Metabolizing Genes Suggests a New Hypothesis Explaining Disease Initiation and Progression. *Life* **2021**, *11*, 886. [CrossRef]
6. Zhang, H.; Wang, L.; Chu, Y. Reactive oxygen species: The signal regulator of B cell. *Free. Radic. Biol. Med.* **2019**, *142*, 16–22. [CrossRef]
7. Cecilia, O.-M.; Alberto, C.-G.J.; Josй, N.-P.; Germбn, C.-M.E.; Karen, L.-C.A.; Miguel, R.-P.L.; Raъl, R.-R.R.; Daniel, R.-C.A. Oxidative Stress as the Main Target in Diabetic Retinopathy Pathophysiology. *J. Diabetes Res.* **2019**, *2019*, 8562408. [CrossRef] [PubMed]
8. Irazabal, M.V.; Torres, V.E. Reactive Oxygen Species and Redox Signaling in Chronic Kidney Disease. *Cells* **2020**, *9*, 1342. [CrossRef] [PubMed]
9. Kang, Q.; Yang, C. Oxidative stress and diabetic retinopathy: Molecular mechanisms, pathogenetic role and therapeutic implications. *Redox Biol.* **2020**, *37*, 101799. [CrossRef]
10. Magnani, F.; Mattevi, A. Structure and mechanisms of ROS generation by NADPH oxidases. *Curr. Opin. Struct. Biol.* **2019**, *59*, 91–97. [CrossRef]
11. Palma, F.R.; He, C.; Danes, J.M.; Paviani, V.; Coelho, D.R.; Gantner, B.N.; Bonini, M.G. Mitochondrial Superoxide Dismutase: What the Established, the Intriguing, and the Novel Reveal About a Key Cellular Redox Switch. *Antioxid. Redox Signal.* **2020**, *32*, 701–714. [CrossRef]
12. Sies, H.; Jones, D.P. Reactive oxygen species (ROS) as pleiotropic physiological signalling agents. *Nat. Rev. Mol. Cell Biol.* **2020**, *21*, 363–383. [CrossRef] [PubMed]
13. Sies, H.; Belousov, V.V.; Chandel, N.S.; Davies, M.J.; Jones, D.P.; Mann, G.E.; Murphy, M.P.; Yamamoto, M.; Winterbourn, C. Defining roles of specific reactive oxygen species (ROS) in cell biology and physiology. *Nat. Rev. Mol. Cell Biol.* **2022**, *23*, 499–515. [CrossRef] [PubMed]
14. Lin, H.-Y.; Weng, S.-W.; Chang, Y.-H.; Su, Y.-J.; Chang, C.-M.; Tsai, C.-J.; Shen, F.-C.; Chuang, J.-H.; Lin, T.-K.; Liou, C.-W.; et al. The Causal Role of Mitochondrial Dynamics in Regulating Insulin Resistance in Diabetes: Link through Mitochondrial Reactive Oxygen Species. *Oxidative Med. Cell. Longev.* **2018**, *2018*, 7514383. [CrossRef]
15. Ahmed, B.; Sultana, R.; Greene, M.W. Adipose tissue and insulin resistance in obese. *Biomed. Pharmacother.* **2021**, *137*, 111315. [CrossRef]
16. Sun, T.; Han, X. Death versus dedifferentiation: The molecular bases of beta cell mass reduction in type 2 diabetes. *Semin. Cell Dev. Biol.* **2020**, *103*, 76–82. [CrossRef] [PubMed]
17. Vermot, A.; Petit-Hдrtlein, I.; Smith, S.; Fieschi, F. NADPH Oxidases (NOX): An Overview from Discovery, Molecular Mechanisms to Physiology and Pathology. *Antioxidants* **2021**, *10*, 890. [CrossRef]
18. Kowluru, R.A.; Mishra, M. Oxidative stress, mitochondrial damage and diabetic retinopathy. *Biochim. Biophys. Acta (BBA)-Mol. Basis Dis.* **2015**, *1852*, 2474–2483. [CrossRef]
19. Kowluru, R.A.; Radhakrishnan, R.; Mohammad, G. Regulation of Rac1 transcription by histone and DNA methylation in diabetic retinopathy. *Sci. Rep.* **2021**, *11*, 14097. [CrossRef]
20. Azarova, I.; Klyosova, E.; Polonikov, A. Association between RAC1 gene variation, redox homeostasis and type 2 diabetes mellitus. *Eur. J. Clin. Investig.* **2022**, *52*, e13792. [CrossRef]
21. World Health Organization. *Definition, Diagnosis, and Classification of Diabetes Mellitus and Its Complications: Report of a WHO Consultation. Part 1: Diagnosis and Classification of Diabetes Mellitus (WHO/NCD/NCS/99.2)*; World Health Organization: Geneva, Switzerland, 1999.
22. World Health Organization. *Use of Glycated Haemoglobin (HbA1c) in the Diagnosis of Diabetes Mellitus. Abbreviated Report of a WHO Consultation (WHO/NMH/CHP/CPM/11.1)*; World Health Organization: Geneva, Switzerland, 2011.

23. Validity of a brief screener for environmental risk factors of age-related diseases using type 2 diabetes and coronary artery disease as examples. *Res. RESULTS Biomed.* **2022**, *8*, 130–137. [CrossRef]
24. Solй, X.; Guiny, E.; Valls, J.; Iniesta, R.; Moreno, V. SNPStats: A web tool for the analysis of association studies. *Bioinformatics* **2006**, *22*, 1928–1929. [CrossRef]
25. Smith, N.L.; Hindorff, L.A.; Heckbert, S.R.; Lemaitre, R.N.; Marciante, K.D.; Rice, K.; Lumley, T.; Bis, J.C.; Wiggins, K.L.; Rosendaal, F.R.; et al. Association of Genetic Variations With Nonfatal Venous Thrombosis in Postmenopausal Women. *JAMA* **2007**, *297*, 489–498. [CrossRef] [PubMed]
26. Shin, S.; Hudson, R.; Harrison, C.; Craven, M.; Keleş, S. atSNP Search: A web resource for statistically evaluating influence of human genetic variation on transcription factor binding. *Bioinformatics* **2019**, *35*, 2657–2659. [CrossRef] [PubMed]
27. Szklarczyk, D.; Gable, A.L.; Nastou, K.C.; Lyon, D.; Kirsch, R.; Pyysalo, S.; Doncheva, N.T.; Legeay, M.; Fang, T.; Bork, P.; et al. The STRING database in 2021: Customizable protein–protein networks, and functional characterization of user-uploaded gene/measurement sets. *Nucleic Acids Res.* **2021**, *49*, D605–D612. [CrossRef] [PubMed]
28. Kashihara, N.; Haruna, Y.; Kondeti, V.K.; Kanwar, Y.S. Oxidative Stress in Diabetic Nephropathy. *Curr. Med. Chem.* **2010**, *17*, 4256–4269. [CrossRef] [PubMed]
29. Pitocco, D.; Tesauro, M.; Alessandro, R.; Ghirlanda, G.; Cardillo, C. Oxidative Stress in Diabetes: Implications for Vascular and Other Complications. *Int. J. Mol. Sci.* **2013**, *14*, 21525–21550. [CrossRef]
30. Tiwari, B.K.; Pandey, K.B.; Abidi, A.B.; Rizvi, S.I. Markers of Oxidative Stress during Diabetes Mellitus. *J. Biomark.* **2013**, *2013*, 378790. [CrossRef]
31. Kowluru, R.A.; Chan, P.S. Oxidative stress and diabetic retinopathy. *Exp Diabetes Res.* **2007**, *2007*, 43603. [CrossRef]
32. Deng, L.; Du, C.; Song, P.; Chen, T.; Rui, S.; Armstrong, D.G.; Deng, W. The Role of Oxidative Stress and Antioxidants in Diabetic Wound Healing. *Oxidative Med. Cell. Longev.* **2021**, *2021*, 8852759. [CrossRef]
33. Antonetti, D.A.; Silva, P.S.; Stitt, A.W. Current understanding of the molecular and cellular pathology of diabetic retinopathy. *Nat. Rev. Endocrinol.* **2021**, *17*, 195–206. [CrossRef]
34. Altmann, C.; Schmidt, M.H. The Role of Microglia in Diabetic Retinopathy: Inflammation, Microvasculature Defects and Neurodegeneration. *Int. J. Mol. Sci.* **2018**, *19*, 110. [CrossRef]
35. Klein, R. *Diabetic Retinopathy Ch.*, 3rd ed.; Duh, E., Ed.; Humana: Louisville, KY, USA, 2008; pp. 67–107.
36. Stitt, A.W.; Curtis, T.M.; Chen, M.; Medina, R.J.; McKay, G.J.; Jenkins, A.; Gardiner, T.A.; Lyons, T.J.; Hammes, H.-P.; Simy, R.; et al. The progress in understanding and treatment of diabetic retinopathy. *Prog. Retin. Eye Res.* **2016**, *51*, 156–186. [CrossRef]
37. Alka, K.; Mohammad, G.; Kowluru, R.A. Regulation of serine palmitoyl-transferase and Rac1–Nox2 signaling in diabetic retinopathy. *Sci. Rep.* **2022**, *12*, 16740. [CrossRef] [PubMed]
38. Sasaki, M.; Ozawa, Y.; Kurihara, T.; Kubota, S.; Yuki, K.; Noda, K.; Kobayashi, S.; Ishida, S.; Tsubota, K. Neurodegenerative influence of oxidative stress in the retina of a murine model of diabetes. *Diabetologia* **2010**, *53*, 971–979. [CrossRef] [PubMed]
39. Wang, W.; Lo, A.C.Y. Diabetic Retinopathy: Pathophysiology and Treatments. *Int. J. Mol. Sci.* **2018**, *19*, 1816. [CrossRef] [PubMed]
40. Selby, N.M.; Taal, M.W. An updated overview of diabetic nephropathy: Diagnosis, prognosis, treatment goals and latest guidelines. *Diabetes, Obes. Metab.* **2020**, *22*, 3–15. [CrossRef]
41. Kopel, J.; Pena-Hernandez, C.; Nugent, K. Evolving spectrum of diabetic nephropathy. *World J. Diabetes* **2019**, *10*, 269–279. [CrossRef]
42. Samsu, N. Diabetic Nephropathy: Challenges in Pathogenesis, Diagnosis, and Treatment. *BioMed Res. Int.* **2021**, *2021*, 16740. [CrossRef]
43. Nishikawa, T.; Edelstein, D.; Du, X.L.; Yamagishi, S.-I.; Matsumura, T.; Kaneda, Y.; Yorek, M.A.; Beebe, D.J.; Oates, P.J.; Hammes, H.-P.; et al. Normalizing mitochondrial superoxide production blocks three pathways of hyperglycaemic damage. *Nature* **2000**, *404*, 787–790. [CrossRef]
44. Tavafi, M. Diabetic nephropathy and antioxidants. *J. Nephropathol.* **2013**, *2*, 20–27. [CrossRef]
45. Donate-Correa, J.; Luis-Rodrнguez, D.; Martнn-Nъcez, E.; Tagua, V.G.; Hern6ndez-Carballo, C.; Ferri, C.; Rodrнguez-Rodrнguez, A.E.; Mora-Fern6ndez, C.; Navarro-Gonz6lez, J.F. Inflammatory Targets in Diabetic Nephropathy. *J. Clin. Med.* **2020**, *9*, 458. [CrossRef] [PubMed]
46. Thallas-Bonke, V.; Thorpe, S.R.; Coughlan, M.T.; Fukami, K.; Yap, F.Y.; Sourris, K.C.; Penfold, S.A.; Bach, L.A.; Cooper, M.E.; Forbes, J.M. Inhibition of NADPH Oxidase Prevents Advanced Glycation End Product–Mediated Damage in Diabetic Nephropathy Through a Protein Kinase C-α–Dependent Pathway. *Diabetes* **2008**, *57*, 460–469. [CrossRef] [PubMed]
47. Hojs, N.V.; Bevc, S.; Ekart, R.; Hojs, R. Oxidative Stress Markers in Chronic Kidney Disease with Emphasis on Diabetic Nephropathy. *Antioxidants* **2020**, *9*, 925. [CrossRef]
48. Cao, Y.; Yang, Z.; Chen, Y.; Jiang, S.; Wu, Z.; Ding, B.; Yang, Y.; Jin, Z.; Tang, H. An Overview of the Posttranslational Modifications and Related Molecular Mechanisms in Diabetic Nephropathy. *Front. Cell Dev. Biol.* **2021**, *9*, 630401. [CrossRef]
49. Hong, Y.; Park, C. Catalytic Antioxidants in the Kidney. *Antioxidants* **2021**, *10*, 130. [CrossRef] [PubMed]
50. Duni, A.; Liakopoulos, V.; Roumeliotis, S.; Peschos, D.; Dounousi, E. Oxidative Stress in the Pathogenesis and Evolution of Chronic Kidney Disease: Untangling Ariadne's Thread. *Int. J. Mol. Sci.* **2019**, *20*, 3711. [CrossRef]
51. Krishan, P.; Chakkarwar, V.A. Diabetic nephropathy: Aggressive involvement of oxidative stress. *J. Pharm. Educ. Res.* **2011**, *2*, 35.
52. Butkowski, E.G.; Jelinek, H.F. Hyperglycaemia, oxidative stress and inflammatory markers. *Redox. Rep.* **2017**, *22*, 257–264. [CrossRef]

53. Lindblom, R.; Higgins, G.; Coughlan, M.; de Haan, J.B. Targeting Mitochondria and Reactive Oxygen Species-Driven Pathogenesis in Diabetic Nephropathy. *Rev. Diabet. Stud.* **2015**, *12*, 134–156. [CrossRef]
54. Chang, A.S.; Hathaway, C.K.; Smithies, O.; Kakoki, M.; Pirklbauer, M.; Schupart, R.; Fuchs, L.; Staudinger, P.; Corazza, U.; Sallaberger, S.; et al. Transforming growth factor-β1 and diabetic nephropathy. *Am. J. Physiol. Physiol.* **2016**, *310*, F689–F696. [CrossRef]
55. Victor, P.; Umapathy, D.; George, L.; Juttada, U.; Ganesh, G.V.; Amin, K.N.; Viswanathan, V.; Ramkumar, K.M. Crosstalk between endoplasmic reticulum stress and oxidative stress in the progression of diabetic nephropathy. *Cell Stress Chaperon.* **2021**, *26*, 311–321. [CrossRef] [PubMed]
56. Warren, A.; Knudsen, S.T.; Cooper, M.E. Diabetic nephropathy: An insight into molecular mechanisms and emerging therapies. *Expert Opin. Ther. Targets* **2019**, *23*, 579–591. [CrossRef] [PubMed]
57. Li, B.; Ye, S.; Fan, Y.; Lin, Y.; Li, S.; Peng, H.; Diao, H.; Chen, W. Identification of novel key genes and potential candidate small molecule drugs in diabetic kidney disease using comprehensive bioinformatics analysis. *Front. Genet.* **2022**, *13*, 934555. [CrossRef] [PubMed]
58. Rico-Fontalvo, J.; Aroca, G.; Cabrales, J.; Daza-Arnedo, R.; Yбnez-Rodrнguez, T.; Martнnez-Бvila, M.C.; Uparella-Gulfo, I.; Raad-Sarabia, M. Molecular Mechanisms of Diabetic Kidney Disease. *Int. J. Mol. Sci.* **2022**, *23*, 8668. [CrossRef]
59. Menne, J.; Shushakova, N.; Bartels, J.; Kiyan, Y.; Laudeley, R.; Haller, H.; Park, J.-K.; Meier, M. Dual Inhibition of Classical Protein Kinase C-α and Protein Kinase C-β Isoforms Protects Against Experimental Murine Diabetic Nephropathy. *Diabetes* **2013**, *62*, 1167–1174. [CrossRef]
60. Vaziri, N.D.; Rodrнguez-Iturbe, B. Mechanisms of Disease: Oxidative stress and inflammation in the pathogenesis of hypertension. *Nat. Clin. Pract. Nephrol.* **2006**, *2*, 582–593. [CrossRef]
61. Burgos-Moryn, E.; Abad-Jimйnez, Z.; de Maracyn, A.M.; Iannantuoni, F.; Lypez, E.; Lypez-Domнnech, S.; Salom, C.; Jover, A.; Mora, V.; Roldan, I.; et al. Relationship between Oxidative Stress, ER Stress, and Inflammation in Type 2 Diabetes: The Battle Continues. *J. Clin. Med.* **2019**, *8*, 1385. [CrossRef]
62. Etoh, T.; Inoguchi, T.; Kakimoto, M.; Sonoda, N.; Kobayashi, K.; Kuroda, J.; Sumimoto, H.; Nawata, H. Increased expression of NAD(P)H oxidase subunits, NOX4 and p22phox, in the kidney of streptozotocin-induced diabetic rats and its reversibity by interventive insulin treatment. *Diabetologia* **2003**, *46*, 1428–1437. [CrossRef]
63. Sedeek, M.; Callera, G.; Montezano, A.; Gutsol, A.; Heitz, F.; Szyndralewiez, C.; Page, P.; Kennedy, C.R.J.; Burns, K.D.; Touyz, R.M.; et al. Critical role of Nox4-based NADPH oxidase in glucose-induced oxidative stress in the kidney: Implications in type 2 diabetic nephropathy. *Am. J. Physiol. Physiol.* **2010**, *299*, F1348–F1358. [CrossRef]
64. Jha, J.C.; Gray, S.P.; Barit, D.; Okabe, J.; El-Osta, A.; Namikoshi, T.; Thallas-Bonke, V.; Wingler, K.; Szyndralewiez, C.; Heitz, F.; et al. Genetic Targeting or Pharmacologic Inhibition of NADPH Oxidase Nox4 Provides Renoprotection in Long-Term Diabetic Nephropathy. *J. Am. Soc. Nephrol.* **2014**, *25*, 1237–1254. [CrossRef] [PubMed]
65. Ying, C.; Zhou, Z.; Dai, J.; Wang, M.; Xiang, J.; Sun, D.; Zhou, X. Activation of the NLRP3 inflammasome by RAC1 mediates a new mechanism in diabetic nephropathy. *Inflamm. Res.* **2022**, *71*, 191–204. [CrossRef] [PubMed]
66. Mokini, Z.; Marcovecchio, M.L.; Chiarelli, F. Molecular pathology of oxidative stress in diabetic angiopathy: Role of mitochondrial and cellular pathways. *Diabetes Res. Clin. Pract.* **2010**, *87*, 313–321. [CrossRef] [PubMed]
67. Folli, F.; Corradi, D.; Fanti, P.; Davalli, A.; Paez, A.; Giaccari, A.; Perego, C.; Muscogiuri, G. The Role of Oxidative Stress in the Pathogenesis of Type 2 Diabetes Mellitus Micro- and Macrovascular Complications: Avenues for a Mechanistic-Based Therapeutic Approach. *Curr. Diabetes Rev.* **2011**, *7*, 313–324. [CrossRef] [PubMed]
68. Xiang, H.; Song, R.; Ouyang, J.; Zhu, R.; Shu, Z.; Liu, Y.; Wang, X.; Zhang, D.; Zhao, J.; Lu, H. Organelle dynamics of endothelial mitochondria in diabetic angiopathy. *Eur. J. Pharmacol.* **2021**, *895*, 173865. [CrossRef]
69. Meza, C.A.; La Favor, J.D.; Kim, D.-H.; Hickner, R.C. Endothelial Dysfunction: Is There a Hyperglycemia-Induced Imbalance of NOX and NOS? *Int. J. Mol. Sci.* **2019**, *20*, 3775. [CrossRef]
70. Suresh, V.; Reddy, A. Dysregulation of nitric oxide synthases during early and late pathophysiological conditions of diabetes mellitus leads to amassing of microvascular impedement. *J. Diabetes Metab. Disord.* **2021**, *20*, 989–1002. [CrossRef]
71. He, T.; Xiong, J.; Nie, L.; Yu, Y.; Guan, X.; Xu, X.; Xiao, T.; Yang, K.; Liu, L.; Zhang, D.; et al. Resveratrol inhibits renal interstitial fibrosis in diabetic nephropathy by regulating AMPK/NOX4/ROS pathway. *J. Mol. Med.* **2016**, *94*, 1359–1371. [CrossRef]
72. Feldman, E.L.; Callaghan, B.C.; Pop-Busui, R.; Zochodne, D.W.; Wright, D.E.; Bennett, D.L.; Bril, V.; Russell, J.W.; Viswanathan, V. Diabetic neuropathy. *Nat. Rev. Dis. Prim.* **2019**, *5*, 41. [CrossRef]
73. Sloan, G.; Selvarajah, D.; Tesfaye, S. Pathogenesis, diagnosis and clinical management of diabetic sensorimotor peripheral neuropathy. *Nat. Rev. Endocrinol.* **2021**, *17*, 400–420. [CrossRef]
74. Casadei, G.; Filippini, M.; Brognara, L. Glycated Hemoglobin (HbA1c) as a Biomarker for Diabetic Foot Peripheral Neuropathy. *Diseases* **2021**, *9*, 16. [CrossRef] [PubMed]
75. Raputova, J.; Srotova, I.; Vlckova, E.; Sommer, C.; Ьзeyler, N.; Birklein, F.; Rittner, H.L.; Rebhorn, C.; Adamova, B.; Kovalova, I.; et al. Sensory phenotype and risk factors for painful diabetic neuropathy: A cross-sectional observational study. *Pain* **2017**, *158*, 2340–2353. [CrossRef] [PubMed]
76. Brownlee, M. The Pathobiology of Diabetic Complications. *Diabetes* **2005**, *54*, 1615–1625. [CrossRef] [PubMed]
77. Iacobini, C.; Vitale, M.; Pesce, C.; Pugliese, G.; Menini, S. Diabetic Complications and Oxidative Stress: A 20-Year Voyage Back in Time and Back to the Future. *Antioxidants* **2021**, *10*, 727. [CrossRef]

78. Figueroa-Romero, C.; Sadidi, M.; Feldman, E.L. Mechanisms of disease: The oxidative stress theory of diabetic neuropathy. *Rev. Endocr. Metab. Disord.* **2008**, *9*, 301–314. [CrossRef]
79. Singh, R.; Kishore, L.; Kaur, N. Diabetic peripheral neuropathy: Current perspective and future directions. *Pharmacol. Res.* **2014**, *80*, 21–35. [CrossRef]
80. Morales, J.; Li, L.; Fattah, F.J.; Dong, Y.; Bey, E.A.; Patel, M.; Gao, J.; Boothman, D.A. Review of Poly (ADP-ribose) Polymerase (PARP) Mechanisms of Action and Rationale for Targeting in Cancer and Other Diseases. *Crit. Rev. Eukaryot. Gene Expr.* **2014**, *24*, 15–28. [CrossRef]
81. Obrosova, I.G.; Drel, V.R.; Pacher, P.; Ilnytska, O.; Wang, Z.Q.; Stevens, M.J.; Yorek, M.A. Oxidative-Nitrosative Stress and Poly(ADP-Ribose) Polymerase (PARP) Activation in Experimental Diabetic Neuropathy. *Diabetes* **2005**, *54*, 3435–3441. [CrossRef]
82. Luna, R.; Manjunatha, R.T.; Bollu, B.; Jhaveri, S.; Avanthika, C.; Reddy, N.; Saha, T.; Gandhi, F. A Comprehensive Review of Neuronal Changes in Diabetics. *Cureus* **2021**, *13*, e19142. [CrossRef]
83. Hernandez-Cardoso, G.G.; Amador-Medina, L.F.; Gutierrez-Torres, G.; Reyes-Reyes, E.S.; Martнnez, C.A.B.; Espinoza, C.C.; Cruz, J.A.; Salas-Gutierrez, I.; Murillo-Ortнz, B.O.; Castro-Camus, E. Terahertz imaging demonstrates its diagnostic potential and reveals a relationship between cutaneous dehydration and neuropathy for diabetic foot syndrome patients. *Sci. Rep.* **2022**, *12*, 3110. [CrossRef]
84. Volmer-Thole, M.; Lobmann, R. Neuropathy and Diabetic Foot Syndrome. *Int. J. Mol. Sci.* **2016**, *17*, 917. [CrossRef]
85. Rossboth, S.; Lechleitner, M.; Oberaigner, W. Risk factors for diabetic foot complications in type 2 diabetes—A systematic review. *Endocrinol. Diabetes Metab.* **2020**, *4*, e00175. [CrossRef]
86. Stancu, B.; Ilyйs, T.; Farcas, M.; Coman, H.F.; Chiș, B.A.; Andercou, O.A. Diabetic Foot Complications: A Retrospective Cohort Study. *Int. J. Environ. Res. Public Health* **2022**, *20*, 187. [CrossRef]
87. Mariadoss, A.V.A.; Sivakumar, A.S.; Lee, C.-H.; Kim, S.J. Diabetes mellitus and diabetic foot ulcer: Etiology, biochemical and molecular based treatment strategies via gene and nanotherapy. *Biomed. Pharmacother.* **2022**, *151*, 129–136. [CrossRef] [PubMed]
88. Qian, J.; Haq, Z.; Yang, D.; Stewart, J.M. Male sex increases the risk of diabetic retinopathy in an urban safety-net hospital population without impacting the relationship between axial length and retinopathy. *Sci. Rep.* **2022**, *12*, 9780. [CrossRef] [PubMed]
89. Liu, L.Y.; Schaub, M.A.; Sirota, M.; Butte, A.J. Sex differences in disease risk from reported genome-wide association study findings. *Hum. Genet.* **2012**, *131*, 353–364. [CrossRef]
90. Randall, J.C.; Winkler, T.W.; Kutalik, Z.; Berndt, S.I.; Jackson, A.U.; Monda, K.L.; Kilpelдinen, T.O.; Esko, T.; Mдgi, R.; Li, S.; et al. Sex-stratified Genome-wide Association Studies Including 270,000 Individuals Show Sexual Dimorphism in Genetic Loci for Anthropometric Traits. *PLoS Genet.* **2013**, *9*, e1003500. [CrossRef] [PubMed]

biomedicines

MDPI

Article

Predictors and Outcomes of SGLT2 Inhibitor Discontinuation in a Real-World Population after Hospitalization for Heart Failure

Masaki Nakagaito, Teruhiko Imamura *, Ryuichi Ushijima, Makiko Nakamura and Koichiro Kinugawa

Second Department of Internal Medicine, University of Toyama, Toyama 930-0152, Japan
* Correspondence: teimamu@med.u-toyama.ac.jp; Tel.: +81-76-434-2281

Abstract: Background: Sodium–glucose cotransporter 2 inhibitors (SGLT2i) reduce mortality and morbidity in patients with heart failure (HF), but are discontinued in some patients. Such patients may not enjoy favorable benefits of SGLT2i therapy. We evaluated the risk factors for SGLT2i discontinuation in a real-world population with HF. Methods: We retrospectively included consecutive patients who were hospitalized for HF and administered SGLT2i during the index hospitalization between February 2016 and September 2021. We assessed the baseline clinical factors associated with post-discharge discontinuation of SGLT2i. Results: This study included a total of 159 patients (median age = 73 years, 57 women). Among baseline characteristics, a lower serum albumin level (odds ratio = 0.23, 95% confidence interval = 0.07–0.76, $p = 0.016$) and a higher dose of furosemide (odds ratio = 1.02, 95% confidence interval = 1.00–1.05, $p = 0.046$) were independently associated with the future discontinuation of SGLT2i following index discharge. Patients who terminated SGLT2i ($n = 19$) had a higher incidence of HF recurrence or cardiovascular death during the 1-year therapeutic period (32% versus 11%, $p = 0.020$). Conclusions: Among patients who initiated SGLT2i during hospitalization for HF, lower serum albumin levels and higher doses of loop diuretic at index discharge were associated with the discontinuation of SGLT2i following index discharge. We should pay special attention to patients with such characteristics during the initiation of SGLT2i and during SGLT2i therapy.

Keywords: cardiovascular disease; heart failure; chronic complications; type 2 diabetes

1. Introduction

To date, sodium–glucose cotransporter 2 inhibitors (SGLT2i) have demonstrated a major therapeutic advance in patients with heart failure (HF). Large-scale randomized controlled trials (RCTs) have shown that they reduce the risk of hospitalization for HF or cardiovascular death in patients with HF with reduced left ventricular ejection fraction (HFrEF) [1,2]. Thus, dapagliflozin and empagliflozin, an example of SGLT2i, have received a class I indication for HFrEF patients in international guidelines [3,4]. The EMPEROR-Preserved trial with empagliflozin and DELIVER trial with dapagliflozin have shown a reduction in HF hospitalization in patients with HF with preserved left ventricular ejection fraction (HFpEF) [5,6]. Furthermore, a reduction in HF hospitalization was reported in patients with HF, independently of the presence of diabetes mellitus (DM). Thus, SGLT2i are prescribed in patients with chronic HF accompanying a wide range of values of left ventricular ejection fraction (LVEF). Recently, several RCTs suggested that SGLT2i might exert a beneficial effect on the cardiovascular outcome even in hospitalized or recently discharged patients with HF, in addition to those with chronic HF [7–9].

However, our team previously found that some studies that initiated SGLT2i terminated SGLT2i for a variety of reasons [10,11]. Patients who terminated SGLT2i had worse clinical outcomes compared with those who continued SGLT2i. Thus, we should pay attention to the negative aspect of SGLT2i therapy. Given their pleiotropic effect, several adverse drug reactions including genital and urinary tract infection [12], volume depletion [13], diabetic ketoacidosis (DKA) [14], bone fractures [15], and amputation [16] might be increased.

Previous large-scale RCTs demonstrated that there was no notable excess of serious treatment-emergent adverse events during SGLT2i therapy. Nevertheless, minor adverse effects of SGLT2i treatment are potentially numerous, and real-world data that reflect actual practice should be useful in identifying them. Of note, although clinical implication of early administration of SGLT2i was investigated in several RCTs including the SOLOIST-WHF trial and EMPULSE trial, whether early-administered SGLT2i can be continued over a longer observational period remains uncertain.

An abundant number of comorbidities including HF and other baseline characteristics may affect the extent of SGLT2i treatment and disturb continuation of SGLT2i therapy. Such risk factors associated with the termination of SGLT2i are of great importance for clinicians in determining whether to initiate SGLT2i and managing patients receiving SGLT2i over a long-term therapeutic period. In the present study, we investigated the factors associated with post-discharge discontinuation of SGLT2i, which was initiated during index hospitalization soon after the stabilization of HF.

2. Materials and Methods

This was a single-center, retrospective observational study to investigate the baseline factors associated with the discontinuation of SGLT2i, which was initiated during index hospitalization. This study was carried out in accordance with the principles outlined in the Declaration of Helsinki, and the institutional ethics board of Toyama University Hospital approved the study protocol (#R2015154, approval date 11 April 2016). Written informed consent was obtained from all of the participants beforehand.

2.1. Study Population

Patients who had been admitted for HF, which was diagnosed according to the Framingham criteria, at our institute between April 2016 and September 2021 were included in this study. Most of the patients had New York Heart Association (NYHA) class III/IV symptoms upon admission. All patients were treated with guideline directed medical therapy for HF, including renin–angiotensin system inhibitors or angiotensin receptor–neprilysin inhibitors, beta-blockers, mineralocorticoid receptor antagonists, and diuretics, if applicable. Patients who newly received SGLT2i during their index hospitalization immediately following the stabilization of hemodynamics were followed-up for 12 months following index discharge (defined as day 0).

2.2. Exclusion Criteria

We excluded the following patients: age < 20 years, end-stage renal failure with estimated glomerular filtration rate (eGFR) < 15 mL/min/1.73 m^2, use of durable left ventricular assist devices, pregnancy or breastfeeding, and current use of SGLT2i during index hospitalization. Patients who stopped taking SGLT2i during index hospitalization were excluded. Adjustment of medical therapy was permitted as a real-world clinical practice. Patients who were lost to follow-up during the 12-month observational period were also excluded. Patients who died due to non-cardiovascular disease were excluded.

2.3. Study Design and Data Collection

Baseline characteristics including demographics and laboratory data at index discharge were retrieved. The eGFR was calculated using the guidelines from the Chronic Kidney Disease Epidemiology Collaboration. Plasma B-type natriuretic peptide (BNP) level and eGFR were retrospectively retrieved at the 12-month follow-up. Standard echocardiographic findings during index hospitalization were retrieved. For the present analysis, participants were divided into HFrEF (LVEF < 40%), HfmrEF (LVEF 40–49%), and HfpEF (LVEF $\geq$ 50%) groups. We defined DM as patients satisfying glycated hemoglobin

(HbA1c) $\geq$ 6.5% or receiving antidiabetic treatment. Bacterial infections included symptomatic bacteriuria or cases where bacterial cultures from sources such as blood, urine, or stool were positive. When patients died from cardiovascular causes, they were censored at the time of events.

2.4. Study Endpoints

The primary outcome was a discontinuation of SGLT2i during the 12 months following their index discharge. Baseline characteristics that would significantly affect the primary outcome were investigated. The secondary outcome was the changes in plasma BNP level and eGFR during the observational period.

2.5. Statistical Analyses

Statistical analysis was conducted using JMP® 15.0 (SAS Institute Inc., Cary, NC, USA). The level of significance was set at two-tailed $p < 0.050$. Continuous variables are presented as the median and interquartile range unless specifically stated. Categorical variables are presented as absolute numbers and percentages. The Wilcoxon test was used to compare continuous parameters, and Pearson's χ^2 test was used for comparison of categorical variables.

Univariable and multivariable analyses with logistic regression models were conducted to calculate the adjusted odds ratio to assess the influence of various baseline parameters on the discontinuation of SGLT2i. Variables deemed as significant ($p < 0.050$) in the univariate analyses were enrolled in the multivariate analyses. Time-to-event outcomes were evaluated using Kaplan–Meier estimates and the two treatment groups were compared with the use of log-rank test statistics.

3. Results

3.1. Follow-Up and Patient Characteristics

Totally, 187 patients met the inclusion criteria. Of them, 2 died from non-cardiovascular causes, and 26 patients were lost to follow-up during the observational period. Finally, 159 patients were included in this study (Figure 1).

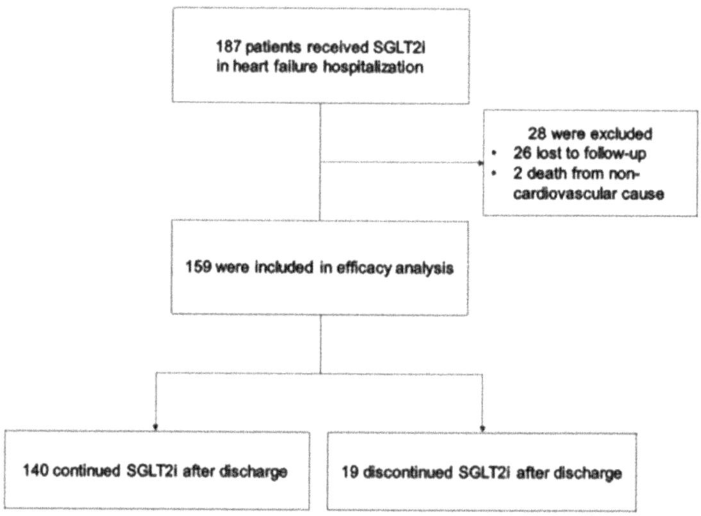

Figure 1. Enrollment and Follow-up.

Table 1 lists the baseline characteristics obtained at index discharge. The median age was 73 (64–81) years and 36% of patients were women. NYHA class III/IV symptoms were noted in 36 patients (23%). HFrEF was noted in 62 patients (39%), HFmrEF in 42 patients

(26%), and HFpEF in 55 patients (35%). DM was noted in 123 patients (77%) (all of them were type 2). As for the types of SGLT2i, 37 patients received canagliflozin, 82 received dapagliflozin, and 40 received empagliflozin. All patients receiving canagliflozin had a history of DM.

Table 1. Baseline characteristics at index discharge.

	Total (n = 159)	Continuation (n = 140)	Discontinuation (n = 19)	p Value
Age, years	73 (64–81)	72 (63–81)	75 (69–83)	0.281
Male, n (%)	102 (64)	93 (66)	9 (47)	0.104
Body weight, kg	57.3 (50.0–66.8)	57.3 (50.2–67.5)	58.7 (47.0–64.1)	0.547
Body mass index, kg/m^2	22.6 (19.8–24.9)	22.6 (19.9–24.9)	22.2 (19.8–23.7)	0.720
Systolic blood pressure, mmHg	105 (96–117)	104 (95–117)	108 (98–118)	0.227
Heart rate, beats per minutes	70 (63–78)	70 (63–78)	71 (65–78)	0.655
Diabetes mellitus, n (%)	123 (77)	105 (75)	18 (95)	0.054
Ischemic etiology, n (%)	66 (42)	58 (41)	8 (42)	0.955
Atrial fibrillation, n (%)	45 (28)	37 (26)	8 (42)	0.155
Implantable cardioverter-defibrillator, n (%)	23 (13)	22 (16)	1 (5)	0.224
Cardiac resynchronization therapy, n (%)	16 (10)	2 (11)	14 (10)	0.943
New York Heart Association class III–IV, n (%)	36 (23)	29 (21)	7 (37)	0.115
Left ventricular ejection fraction, %	43 (33–55)	43 (33–55)	43 (31–60)	0.744
Value of <40% (HFrEF), n (%)	62 (39)	54 (39)	8 (42)	0.767
Value of 40–49% (HFmrEF), n (%)	42 (26)	37 (26)	5 (26)	0.992
Value of ≥50% (HFpEF), n (%)	55 (35)	49 (35)	6 (32)	0.769
HbA1c, %	6.7 (6.4–7.6)	6.7 (6.3–7.6)	6.9 (6.5–7.6)	0.404
Fasting blood sugar, mg/dL	110 (95–132)	110 (95–130)	121 (93–152)	0.230
Hemoglobin, g/dL	12.5 (11.2–13.9)	12.6 (11.2–14.1)	11.9 (10.6–13.5)	0.089
Hematocrit, %	37.8 (34.1–41.4)	38.0 (34.2–41.6)	35.5 (32.2–40.6)	0.135
Serum albumin, g/dL	3.6 (3.4–3.9)	3.7 (3.4–4.0)	3.4 (3.2–3.6)	0.006 *
Serum sodium, mEq/L	138 (136–140)	138 (137–140)	136 (135–140)	0.258
Serum potassium, mEq/L	4.3 (4.1–4.6)	4.3 (4.1–4.6)	4.5 (3.9–4.8)	0.641
eGFR, mL/minute/1.73 m^2	50.5 (36.9–64.4)	51.2 (36.9–66.6)	41.2 (36.9–58.8)	0.342
Uric acid, mg/dL	5.7 (4.8–6.9)	5.7 (4.8–7.0)	6.0 (5.6–6.7)	0.418
Plasma BNP, pg/mL	142 (69–284)	142 (69–269)	182 (68–477)	0.237
Heart failure therapies				
Beta-blockers, n (%)	142 (89)	124 (89)	18 (95)	0.415
ACEI/ARB/ARNI, n (%)	149 (94)	130 (93)	19 (100)	0.229
Loop diuretics, n (%)	102 (64)	88 (63)	14 (74)	0.356
Dose of furosemide, mg/day	10 (0–20)	10 (0–20)	20 (0–20)	0.223
MRA, n (%)	54 (34)	44 (31)	10 (53)	0.067
Thiazides, n (%)	3 (2)	3 (2)	0 (0)	0.520
Anti-diabetic agents				
Sulfonylureas, n (%)	6 (4)	6 (4)	0 (0)	0.358
DPP-4i, n (%)	62 (39)	53 (38)	9 (47)	0.425
Biguanides, n (%)	22 (14)	21 (15)	1 (5)	0.249
Insulin, n (%)	13 (8)	10 (7)	3 (16)	0.197
Sodium–glucose cotransporter 2 inhibitors				
Canagliflozin, n (%)	37 (23)	32 (23)	5 (26)	0.738
Dapagliflozin, n (%)	82 (52)	75 (54)	7 (37)	0.171
Empagliflozin, n (%)	40 (25)	33 (24)	7 (37)	0.211

eGFR, estimated glomerular filtration rate; HFrEF, heart failure with reduced ejection fraction (ejection fraction < 40%); HFmrEF, heart failure with mildly reduced ejection fraction (ejection fraction 40–49%); HFpEF, heart failure with preserved ejection fraction (ejection fraction ≥ 50%); HbA1c, glycated hemoglobin; BNP, B-type natriuretic peptide; NT-proBNP, N-terminal pro-B-type natriuretic peptide; ACEI, angiotensin-converting enzyme inhibitors; ARB, angiotensin receptor blockers; ARNI, angiotensin receptor–neprilysin inhibitors; MRA, mineralocorticoid receptor antagonists; DPP-4i, dipeptidyl peptidase-4 inhibitors. * $p < 0.050$.

3.2. Causes of Primary Outcome

As a primary outcome, a total 19 of patients (12.0%) encountered the discontinuation of SGLT2i. The most common reasons for SGLT2i discontinuation were bacterial infection (n = 6, 32%), followed by patient-reported side effects (n = 5, 26%). The side effects reported by patients included nocturia, anorexia, pruritus, and tiredness. Adjustment for treatment of cardiovascular disease was the third most common reason (n = 4, 21%) (Figure 2).

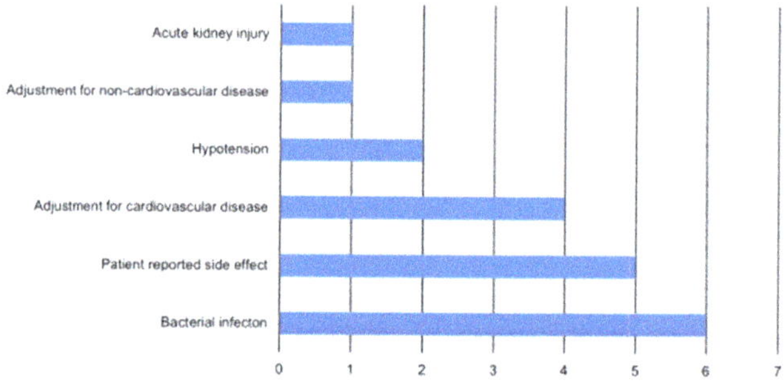

Figure 2. Reasons for discontinuation of SGLT2 inhibitors (n = 19).

3.3. Prediction of Primary Outcome

Baseline characteristics stratified by achievement of primary endpoint are summarized in Table 1. The level of serum albumin was lower in the discontinuation group than the continuation group. Medications for HF and DM were not statistically different between the two groups. There were no significant differences in the plasma BNP and eGFR levels at baseline between both groups.

Univariable and multivariable analyses demonstrated that serum albumin level (odds ratio = 0.23, 95% confidence interval = 0.07–0.76, p = 0.016) was independently and negatively associated with the discontinuation of SGLT2i, and furosemide dosage (odds ratio = 1.02, 95% = confidence interval 1.00–1.05, p = 0.046) was positively associated with the discontinuation of SGLT2i (Table 2). Prevalence of DM was not associated with the primary outcome.

Table 2. Variables associated with discontinuation of SGLT2 inhibitors.

	All Patients (n = 159)					
	Univariable Analysis			Multivariable Analysis		
Variables	Odds Ratio	95% CI	p Value	Odds Ratio	95% CI	p Value
Age, years	1.03	0.98–1.08	0.224			
Male, yes	0.46	0.17–1.20	0.110			
Body mass index, kg/m^2	0.97	0.86–1.10	0.657			
Systolic blood pressure, mmHg	1.02	0.99–1.05	0.136			
Heart rate, bpm	1.01	0.97–1.06	0.578			
Ischemic etiology, yes	1.03	0.39–2.71	0.955			
Atrial fibrillation, yes	2.03	0.73–5.40	0.161			
NYHA class III–IV, n (%)	2.23	0.81–6.18	0.122			
HFrEF, yes	1.16	0.44–3.06	0.767			
Diabetes mellitus, yes	6.00	0.77–46.59	0.087			
Fasting blood sugar, mg/dL	1.01	1.00–1.02	0.219			
Hematocrit, %	0.93	0.85–1.03	0.157			
Serum albumin, g/dL	0.19	0.06–0.62	0.006 *	0.23	0.07–0.76	0.016 *
Serum sodium, mEq/L	0.96	0.84–1.10	0.551			
Serum potassium, mEq/L	1.24	0.47–3.29	0.670			
eGFR, mL/min/1.73 m^2	0.99	0.97–1.02	0.605			
Uric acid, mg/dL	1.07	0.81–1.42	0.638			
ln BNP	1.41	0.85–2.33	0.187			
Beta-blockers, yes	2.32	0.29–18.59	0.427			
ACEI/ARB/ARNI, yes	NA	NA	0.993			
Loop diuretics, yes	1.66	0.56–4.86	0.360			
Dose of furosemide, mg/day	1.03	1.01–1.05	0.013 *	1.02	1.00–1.05	0.046 *
MRA, yes	2.42	0.92–6.39	0.073			
Thiazides, yes	NA	NA	0.991			
Sulfonylureas, yes	NA	NA	0.992			
DPP-4i, yes	1.48	0.56–3.87	0.427			
Biguanides, yes	0.32	0.04–2.49	0.273			
Insulin, yes	2.44	0.61–9.79	0.209			

NYHA, New York Heart Association; HFrEF, heart failure with reduced ejection fraction (ejection fraction < 40%); LVEF, left ventricular ejection fraction; HbA1c, glycated hemoglobin; eGFR, estimated glomerular filtration rate; BNP, B-type natriuretic peptide; ACEI, angiotensin-converting enzyme inhibitors; ARB, angiotensin receptor blockers; ARNI, angiotensin receptor–neprilysin inhibitors; MRA, mineralocorticoid receptor antagonists; NA, not applicable. * p < 0.050.

3.4. Impact of SGLT2i Discontinuation on Clinical Outcomes

Patients in the discontinued SGLT2i group had a higher incidence of recurrent HF hospitalization or cardiovascular death (32% vs. 11%, $p = 0.020$; Figure 3).

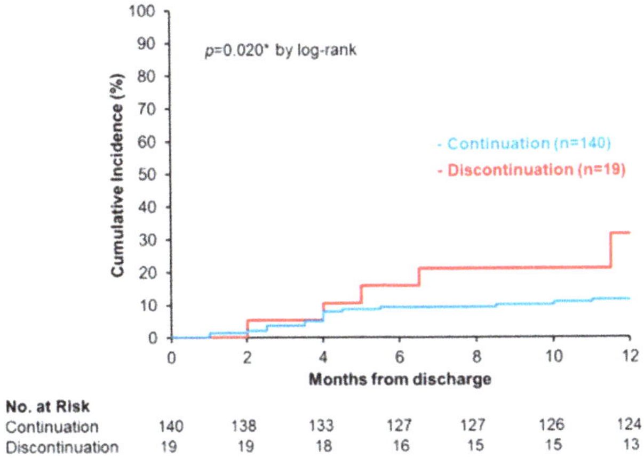

Figure 3. Recurrent hospitalization for heart failure or cardiovascular death in patients with continued SGLT2 inhibitors versus those with discontinued SGLT2 inhibitors. * $p < 0.050$.

The changes in plasma BNP and eGFR were assessed in 117 and 133 patients, respectively, by excluding those who died during the observational period and those whose laboratory data were not retrieved. Changes in plasma BNP level from baseline are shown in Figure 4. Plasma BNP levels decreased in patients with both continuation and discontinuation of SGLT2i from baseline to 12 months. The changes in plasma BNP were not different between the continued SGLT2i group and the discontinued SGLT2i group (−20.5 vs. −96.0 pg/mL, $p = 0.096$). On the other hand, there were no significant changes in eGFR throughout the 12-month observation period in both groups. The changes in eGFR were not different between the continued SGLT2i group and the discontinued SGLT2i group (+0.65 vs. −0.60 mL/min/1.73 m^2, $p = 0.767$).

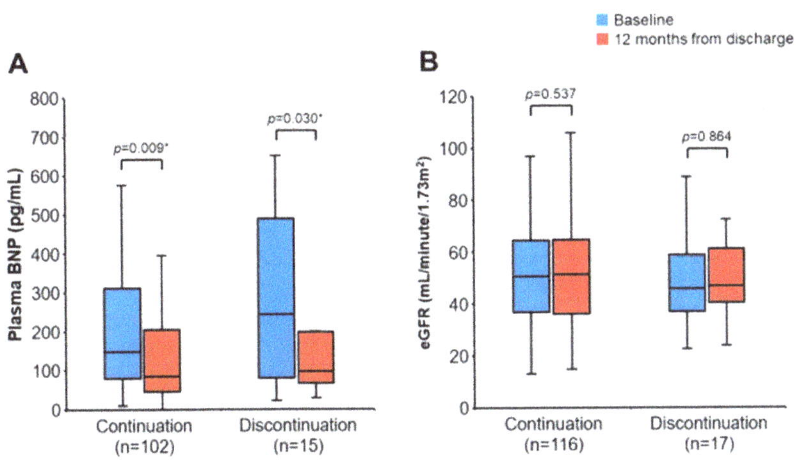

Figure 4. Changes in plasma BNP (**A**) and estimated GFR (**B**) during 12-month observational period following index discharge. Variables were compared by Wilcoxon singed-rank test. * $p < 0.050$.

4. Discussion

We investigated the factors associated with post-discharge discontinuation of SGLT2i in patients with HF. SGLT2i were initiated soon after the stabilization of hemodynamics during index hospitalization for HF. Among baseline characteristics at index discharge, a lower serum albumin level and a higher dose of furosemide were associated with discontinuation of SGLT2i following index discharge. Patients with discontinued SGLT2i had a higher incidence of re-hospitalization for HF or cardiovascular death during the 12-month observational period following index discharge. The changes in plasma BNP and eGFR were not significantly different between the discontinued SGLT2i group and the continued SGLT2i group.

4.1. Discontinuation of SGLT2i

In this study, SGLT2i were discontinued for reasons other than death in 19 patients (12.0%). Our discontinuation rate of 12.0% is similar to previously reported rates of 10.5–23.2% in large-scale RCTs [1,2,5,6]. However, the median follow-up durations of these RCTs (16.0–27.9 months) were longer than ours (12.0 months), and the risk of SGLT2i discontinuation in this study might be higher than in previous RCTs. In the SOLOIST-WHF trial and EMPULSE trial, both of which investigated the clinical implication of early initiation of SGLT2i, the rates of adverse events leading to the discontinuation of SGLT2i were lower than those in the present study (8.5% and 4.8%, respectively) [7,8]. These findings suggest difficulty in continuing SGLT2i in real-world populations.

A possible explanation for the high frequency of SGLT2i discontinuation was that our patients were included in this study soon after an episode of decompensated HF. Our population might be distinct from patients with chronic HF in most of the previous trials, since our patients were at a higher risk of cardiovascular events compared to patients in many of the other trials. Additionally, our population may have a higher risk of SGLT2i withdrawal in the vulnerable period, in which patients may have unstable volume status, renal function, and blood pressure and other HF therapies may require adjustment. Similarly, a subset of the DELIVER trial, which evaluated the response to dapagliflozin in hospitalized or recently discharged patients, reported that serious adverse events were more common in recently hospitalized patients compared with those without episodes of recent hospitalization [17].

4.2. Diabetes and SGLT2i Discontinuation

Importantly, prevalence of DM was no longer a predictor of SGLT2i discontinuation in this study. Further, no patients stopped SGLT2i because of major hypoglycemia or DKA. Our observation regarding the safety of SGLT2i is consistent with previous trials and reports that the rate of SGLT2i discontinuation is not significantly different between participants with and without diabetes.

4.3. Hypoalbuminemia and SGLT2i Discontinuation

We demonstrated that a lower serum albumin level and a higher dose of furosemide were associated with SGLT2i discontinuation. It is worth noting that both low serum albumin levels and high doses of furosemide at baseline are strongly associated with an increased risk of HF [18–20]. In addition, SGLT2i therapy for patients with malnutrition might not be encouraged due to its potential to progress catabolism. Although subsets of the DAPA-HF trial and DELIVER trial demonstrated that dapagliflozin improved cardiovascular outcomes regardless of frailty status [21,22], few studies assessed the efficacy and safety of SGLT2i in malnourished patients. Our finding suggests that caution should be exercised in using SGLT2i in patients with both HF and malnutrition.

4.4. High Dose of Loop Diuretics and SGLT2i Discontinuation

High incidence of SGLT2 discontinuation in patients with high doses of furosemide may be associated with adverse events of volume depletion. Although individual RCTs reported that the frequency of adverse events related to volume depletion did not differ between patients with SGLT2i and those without SGLT2i, a meta-analysis indicated that there is an increase in hypovolemia associated with SGLT2i treatment [13]. Moreover, a previous study reported that SGLT2i therapy resulted in a significant augmentation of natriuresis when combined with loop diuretics [23]. Inhibition of compensatory absorption of sodium in the Henle's loop or distal tubule by loop diuretics in patients receiving SGLT2 may explain the findings of the study.

Therefore, co-administration of SGLT2i and high-dose loop diuretics might act complementarily via double blocking of proximal tubules and Henle's loop, resulting in rapid volume depletion. This diuretic profile offers significant advantages in the management of volume status in patients with HF, whereas a robust diuretic response may result in excessive fluid loss. In this study, unexpected changes in plasma volume caused by co-administration of SGLT2i and high-dose loop diuretics may have led to SGLT2i discontinuation.

4.5. Outcomes of SGLT2i Discontinuation

In our study, patients who discontinued SGLT2i had a higher risk of re-hospitalization for HF or cardiovascular death. This result should be interpreted with caution since this is a retrospective observational study. We found that lower serum albumin levels and higher doses of furosemide were independently associated with SGLT2i discontinuation, and were also associated with an increased risk of HF. Patients who discontinued SGLT2i may be at higher risk of cardiovascular events than those who continued SGLT2i, making it difficult to assess the association between SGLT2i discontinuation and cardiovascular outcome in this study.

On the other hand, we previously reported that patients who discontinued SGLT2i at discharge from hospitalization for HF were more likely to be re-hospitalized for HF than those who continued SGLT2i [11]. Previous findings may support a direct and independent prophylactic effect of SGLT2i on cardiovascular events for post-discharge patients in this study. RCTs demonstrated that SGLT2i improved cardiovascular outcomes, whereas few studies reported the effect of discontinuing SGLT2i on cardiovascular events. Additional research to confirm these findings and to understand the importance of continuing SGLT2i after discharge from hospitalization for HF is needed.

4.6. Limitations

This study has several limitations. First, this study was conducted retrospectively in a single center, and both overall sample size and number of patients reaching the primary outcome were small. Given the low event number, the number of potential confounders included in the multivariate analyses was limited. Similarly, limited patients were included in the analysis for secondary outcome. Furthermore, it is not possible to establish a cause–effect relationship given the retrospective observational study design. Second, other HF medications were also adjusted during the observational period in this study. Thus, it is challenging to assess the effect of SGLT2i alone. Lastly, our population received multiple types of SGLT2i in the present study. No RCTs have evaluated the efficacy of canagliflozin in patients with HF. It remains unclear whether such beneficial effects are consistent across individual SGLT2i. However, a recent retrospective cohort study reported that there was no significant difference in the risk of cardiovascular events including HF among patients taking dapagliflozin, canagliflozin, and empagliflozin [24].

5. Conclusions

In this study, we found that 12.0% of patients who initiated SGLT2i soon after the stabilization of their HF during index hospitalization terminated SGLT2i therapy within 12 months following index discharge. The rate of discontinuation of SGLT2i is slightly higher than those of previous RCTs. The most common reason for the discontinuation of SGLT2i was bacterial infection. Lower serum albumin levels and higher doses of furosemide at the time of index discharge were independently associated with SGLT2 discontinuation after discharge from hospitalization for HF. Furthermore, SGLT2i discontinuation was associated with an increased risk of re-hospitalization for HF or cardiovascular death. Special attention should be paid when initiating and managing SGLT2i for those with such risk factors.

Author Contributions: M.N. (Masaki Nakagaito) wrote the draft. T.I. analyzed and interpreted the patient data. R.U. and M.N. (Makiko Nakamura) collected data and reviewed the draft. K.K. supervised the study. All authors have read and agreed to the published version of the manuscript.

Funding: This research received no external funding.

Institutional Review Board Statement: The study was conducted according to the guidelines of the Declaration of Helsinki and approved by the Institutional Ethics Board of Toyama University Hospital (#R2015154; date of approval: 11 April 2016).

Informed Consent Statement: Informed consent was obtained from all subjects involved in the study.

Data Availability Statement: The data presented in this study are available on request from the corresponding author. The data are not publicly available due to privacy.

Conflicts of Interest: The authors declare no conflict of interest.

References

1. McMurray, J.J.V.; Solomon, S.D.; Inzucchi, S.E.; Køber, L.; Kosiborod, M.N.; Martinez, F.A.; Ponikowski, P.; Sabatine, M.S.; Anand, I.S.; Bělohlávek, J.; et al. Dapagliflozin in Patients with Heart Failure and Reduced Ejection Fraction. *N. Engl. J. Med.* **2019**, *381*, 1995–2008. [CrossRef] [PubMed]
2. Packer, M.; Anker, S.D.; Butler, J.; Filippatos, G.; Pocock, S.J.; Carson, P.; Januzzi, J.; Verma, S.; Tsutsui, H.; Brueckmann, M.; et al. Cardiovascular and Renal Outcomes with Empagliflozin in Heart Failure. *N. Engl. J. Med.* **2020**, *383*, 1413–1424. [CrossRef] [PubMed]
3. Heidenreich, P.A.; Bozkurt, B.; Aguilar, D.; Allen, L.A.; Byun, J.J.; Colvin, M.M.; Deswal, A.; Drazner, M.H.; Dunlay, S.M.; Evers, L.R.; et al. 2022 AHA/ACC/HFSA Guideline for the Management of Heart Failure: A Report of the American College of Cardiology/American Heart Association Joint Committee on Clinical Practice Guidelines. *J. Am. Coll. Cardiol.* **2022**, *79*, e263–e421. [CrossRef]
4. McDonagh, T.A.; Metra, M.; Adamo, M.; Gardner, R.S.; Baumbach, A.; Böhm, M.; Burri, H.; Butler, J.; Čelutkienė, J.; Chioncel, O.; et al. 2021 ESC Guidelines for the diagnosis and treatment of acute and chronic heart failure: Developed by the Task Force for the diagnosis and treatment of acute and chronic heart failure of the European Society of Cardiology (ESC). With the special contribution of the Heart Failure Association (HFA) of the ESC. *Eur. J. Heart Fail.* **2022**, *24*, 4–131. [CrossRef] [PubMed]
5. Anker, S.D.; Butler, J.; Filippatos, G.; Ferreira, J.P.; Bocchi, E.; Böhm, M.; Brunner-La Rocca, H.P.; Choi, D.J.; Chopra, V.; Chuquiure-Valenzuela, E.; et al. Empagliflozin in Heart Failure with a Preserved Ejection Fraction. *N. Engl. J. Med.* **2021**, *385*, 1451–1461. [CrossRef]
6. Solomon, S.D.; McMurray, J.J.V.; Claggett, B.; de Boer, R.A.; DeMets, D.; Hernandez, A.F.; Inzucchi, S.E.; Kosiborod, M.N.; Lam, C.S.P.; Martinez, F.; et al. Dapagliflozin in Heart Failure with Mildly Reduced or Preserved Ejection Fraction. *N. Engl. J. Med.* **2022**, *387*, 1089–1098. [CrossRef]
7. Voors, A.A.; Angermann, C.E.; Teerlink, J.R.; Collins, S.P.; Kosiborod, M.; Biegus, J.; Ferreira, J.P.; Nassif, M.E.; Psotka, M.A.; Tromp, J.; et al. The SGLT2 inhibitor empagliflozin in patients hospitalized for acute heart failure: A multinational randomized trial. *Nat. Med.* **2022**, *28*, 568–574. [CrossRef]
8. Bhatt, D.L.; Szarek, M.; Steg, P.G.; Cannon, C.P.; Leiter, L.A.; McGuire, D.K.; Lewis, J.B.; Riddle, M.C.; Voors, A.A.; Metra, M.; et al. Sotagliflozin in Patients with Diabetes and Recent Worsening Heart Failure. *N. Engl. J. Med.* **2021**, *384*, 117–128. [CrossRef]
9. Schulze, P.C.; Bogoviku, J.; Westphal, J.; Aftanski, P.; Haertel, F.; Grund, S.; von Haehling, S.; Schumacher, U.; Möbius-Winkler, S.; Busch, M. Effects of Early Empagliflozin Initiation on Diuresis and Kidney Function in Patients with Acute Decompensated Heart Failure (EMPAG-HF). *Circulation* **2022**, *146*, 289–298. [CrossRef]
10. Nakagaito, M.; Imamura, T.; Joho, S.; Ushijima, R.; Nakamura, M.; Kinugawa, K. Factors Associated with Recurrent Heart Failure during Incorporating SGLT2 Inhibitors in Patients Hospitalized for Acute Decompensated Heart Failure. *J. Clin. Med.* **2022**, *11*, 5027. [CrossRef]
11. Nakagaito, M.; Imamura, T.; Joho, S.; Ushijima, R.; Nakamura, M.; Kinugawa, K. Efficacy of Continuing SGLT2 Inhibitors on Outcomes in Patients with Acute Decompensated Heart Failure. *Int. Heart J.* **2021**, *62*, 885–890. [CrossRef]
12. Liu, J.; Li, L.; Li, S.; Jia, P.; Deng, K.; Chen, W.; Sun, X. Effects of SGLT2 inhibitors on UTIs and genital infections in type 2 diabetes mellitus: A systematic review and meta-analysis. *Sci. Rep.* **2017**, *7*, 2824. [CrossRef]
13. Rong, X.; Zhu, Y.; Wen, B.; Liu, K.; Li, X.; Gou, Q.; Chen, X. Risk of hypovolemia associated with sodium-glucose cotransporter-2 inhibitors treatment: A meta-analysis of randomized controlled trials. *Front. Cardiovasc. Med.* **2022**, *9*, 973129. [CrossRef]

14. Liu, J.; Li, L.; Li, S.; Wang, Y.; Qin, X.; Deng, K.; Liu, Y.; Zou, K.; Sun, X. Sodium-glucose co-transporter-2 inhibitors and the risk of diabetic ketoacidosis in patients with type 2 diabetes: A systematic review and meta-analysis of randomized controlled trials. *Diabetes Obes. Metab.* **2020**, *22*, 1619–1627. [CrossRef]
15. Adimadhyam, S.; Lee, T.A.; Calip, G.S.; Smith Marsh, D.E.; Layden, B.T.; Schumock, G.T. Sodium-glucose co-transporter 2 inhibitors and the risk of fractures: A propensity score-matched cohort study. *Pharmacoepidemiol. Drug Saf.* **2019**, *28*, 1629–1639. [CrossRef]
16. Khouri, C.; Cracowski, J.L.; Roustit, M. SGLT-2 inhibitors and the risk of lower-limb amputation: Is this a class effect? *Diabetes Obes. Metab.* **2018**, *20*, 1531–1534. [CrossRef]
17. Cunningham, J.W.; Vaduganathan, M.; Claggett, B.L.; Kulac, I.J.; Desai, A.S.; Jhund, P.S.; de Boer, R.A.; DeMets, D.; Hernandez, A.F.; Inzucchi, S.E.; et al. Dapagliflozin in Patients Recently Hospitalized wth Heart Failure and Mildly Reduced or Preserved Ejection Fraction. *J. Am. Coll. Cardiol.* **2022**, *80*, 1302–1310. [CrossRef]
18. Gopal, D.M.; Kalogeropoulos, A.P.; Georgiopoulou, V.V.; Tang, W.W.; Methvin, A.; Smith, A.L.; Bauer, D.C.; Newman, A.B.; Kim, L.; Harris, T.B.; et al. Serum albumin concentration and heart failure risk the Health, Aging, and Body Composition Study. *Am. Heart J.* **2010**, *160*, 279–285. [CrossRef]
19. Uthamalingam, S.; Kandala, J.; Daley, M.; Patvardhan, E.; Capodilupo, R.; Moore, S.A.; Januzzi, J.L., Jr. Serum albumin and mortality in acutely decompensated heart failure. *Am. Heart J.* **2010**, *160*, 1149–1155. [CrossRef]
20. Hasselblad, V.; Gattis Stough, W.; Shah, M.R.; Lokhnygina, Y.; O'Connor, C.M.; Califf, R.M.; Adams, K.F., Jr. Relation between dose of loop diuretics and outcomes in a heart failure population: Results of the ESCAPE trial. *Eur. J. Heart Fail.* **2007**, *9*, 1064–1069. [CrossRef]
21. Butt, J.H.; Dewan, M.P.; Merkely, B.; Belohlávek, J.; Drożdż, J.; Kitakaze, M.; Inzucchi, S.E.; Kosiborod, M.N.; Martinez, F.A.; Tereshchenko, S.; et al. Efficacy and Safety of Dapagliflozin According to Frailty in Heart Failure with Reduced Ejection Fraction: A Post Hoc Analysis of the DAPA-HF Trial. *Ann. Intern. Med.* **2022**, *175*, 820–830. [CrossRef] [PubMed]
22. Butt, J.H.; Jhund, P.S.; Belohlávek, J.; de Boer, R.A.; Chiang, C.-E.; Desai, A.S.; Drożdżż, J.; Hernandez, A.F.; Inzucchi, S.E.; Katova, T.; et al. Efficacy and Safety of Dapagliflozin According to Frailty in Patients with Heart Failure: A Prespecified Analysis of the DELIVER Trial. *Circulation* **2022**, *146*, 1210–1224. [CrossRef] [PubMed]
23. Griffin, M.; Rao, V.S.; Ivey-Miranda, J.; Fleming, J.; Mahoney, D.; Maulion, C.; Suda, N.; Siwakoti, K.; Ahmad, T.; Jacoby, D.; et al. Empagliflozin in Heart Failure: Diuretic and Cardiorenal Effects. *Circulation* **2020**, *142*, 1028–1039. [CrossRef] [PubMed]
24. Suzuki, Y.; Kaneko, H.; Okada, A.; Itoh, H.; Matsuoka, S.; Fujiu, K.; Michihata, N.; Jo, T.; Takeda, N.; Morita, H.; et al. Comparison of cardiovascular outcomes between SGLT2 inhibitors in diabetes mellitus. *Cardiovasc. Diabetol.* **2022**, *21*, 67. [CrossRef] [PubMed]

biomedicines

MDPI

Article

Mitochondrial DNA Polymorphism in HV1 and HV2 Regions and 12S rDNA in Perimenopausal Hypertensive Women

Wojciech Kwaśniewski [1], Aleksandra Stupak [2,*], Alicja Warowicka [3], Anna Goździcka-Józefiak [3], Jerzy Mosiewicz [4] and Jolanta Mieczkowska [4]

1 Gynecology and Oncological Gynecology Department, Medical University of Lublin, 20-081 Lublin, Poland
2 Obstetrics and Pregnancy Pathology Department, Medical University of Lublin, 20-081 Lublin, Poland
3 Department of Molecular Virology, Adam Mickiewicz University in Poznan, 61-712 Poznan, Poland
4 Internal Diseases Department, Medical University of Lublin, 20-081 Lublin, Poland
* Correspondence: aleksandra.stupak@umlub.pl

Abstract: Estrogens enhance cellular mitochondrial activity. The diminution of female hormones during menopause may have an effect on the mitochondrial genome and the expression of mitochondrial proteins. Hence, oxidative stress and the pro-inflammatory state contribute to the formation of systemic illnesses including arterial hypertension (AH). This study aimed to determine the types and frequency of mutations in the mitochondrial DNA (mtDNA) nucleotide sequence in the hypervariable regions 1 and 2 (HV1 and HV2) and the 12S RNA coding sequence of the D-loop in postmenopausal women with hypertension. In our study, 100 women were investigated, 53 of whom were postmenopausal and 47 of whom were premenopausal (53.9 ± 3.7 years vs. 47.7 ± 4.2 years, respectively). Of those studied, 35 premenopausal and 40 postmenopausal women were diagnosed with AH. A medical checkup with 24 h monitoring of blood pressure (RR) and heart rate was undertaken (HR). The polymorphism of the D-loop and 12S rDNA region of mtDNA was examined. Changes in the nucleotide sequence of mtDNA were observed in 23% of the group of 100 women. The changes were identified in 91.3% of HV1 and HV2 regions, 60.9% of HV1 segments, 47.5% of HV2 regions, and 43.5% of 12S rDNA regions. The frequency of nucleotide sequence alterations in mtDNA was substantially higher in postmenopausal women (34%) than in premenopausal women (10.6%), $p = 0.016$. A higher frequency of changes in HV1 + HV2 sections in postmenopausal women (30.2%) compared to the premenopausal group (10.6%) was detected, $p = 0.011$. Only postmenopausal women were found to have modifications to the HV2 segment and the 12S rDNA region. After menopause, polymorphism in the mtDNA region was substantially more frequent in women with arterial hypertension than before menopause ($p = 0.030$; 37.5% vs. 11.5%). Comparable findings were observed in the HV2 and HV1 regions of the AH group (35% vs. 11.5%), $p = 0.015$, in the HV1 segment (25% vs. 11.5%), $p = 0.529$, and in the HV2 segment, 12S rDNA (25% vs. 0%). More than 80% of all changes in nucleotide sequence were homoplasmic. The mtDNA polymorphisms of the nucleotide sequence in the HV1 and HV2 regions, the HV2 region alone, and the 12S RNA coding sequence were associated with estrogen deficiency and a more severe course of arterial hypertension, accompanied by symptoms of adrenergic stimulation.

Keywords: mtDNA; nucleotide sequence; polymorphism; HV1 region; HV2 region; D-loop; menopause; arterial hypertension

1. Background

1.1. Mitochondrial DNA

The research of mitochondrial genome polymorphism began in the 1980s, when new tools in molecular biology made it possible to identify the mtDNA mitochondrial genome sequence [1]. The first mutation in the mitochondrial genome was described in 1988 and involved nucleotide 8344, a shift in the A/G sequence that causes myoclonic epilepsy accompanied with the presence of ragged red fibers in the muscles (MERRF syndrome, myoclonic epilepsy, and ragged red fibers) [2]. In human cells, the genetic material of the mitochondria constitutes 1% of the cell's DNA [3]. MtDNA is a circular molecule containing 16,569 base pairs (bp) and is situated in the matrix of mitochondria. Each mitochondria carries four to ten copies of mtDNA [4,5]. The arrangement and structure of the mitochondrial genome parallels that of the bacterial genome. Moreover, mitochondrial ribosomes are prokaryotic in nature. Histone proteins are absent in mtDNA. Additional proteins related to mitochondrial DNA form structures known as nucleoids (nt). In both strands of mtDNA, 37 genes have been found in the mitochondrial genome (28 on the H (heavy) strand and 9 on the L (light) strand). Genes are tightly packed in mitochondrial DNA, and the sequences of some genes overlap and overlap (ATP8 and ATP6, ND4L, and ND4); there are few non-coding regions [6–10]. Mitochondria are also responsible for apoptosis' so-called internal route. Along with this process is the release of cytochrome c and other proteins from the mitochondria. Released from the mitochondria, cytochrome c contributes to the synthesis of the Apoptosome protein complex [11]. Mitochondrial proteins belonging to the BCL-2 family, which are mostly localized in the outer mitochondrial membrane, and factor or endonuclease G are also implicated in the mitochondrial apoptotic process [12].

1.2. The D-Loop in mtDNA

The D-loop, which comprises 7% of the mitochondrial genome and regulates replication and transcription of mitochondrial genes, is an important non-coding region in mtDNA. It is composed of 1122 base pairs (from 16,024 nt to 567 nt mtDNA) and is located between the genes encoding the tRNA Pro and the tRNA Phe. The nucleotide sequences responsible for initiating gene transcription and mitochondrial genome replication have been found in this area [6,13–15]. In the D-loop region, there are also two hypervariable regions: the first (HV1) from 16,024 nt to 16,383 nt and the second (HV2) from 57 nt to 33 nt. In these places, the nucleotide sequence polymorphism is utilized in forensic investigations and medical diagnostics [16]. Additional variable regions in the D-loop of mtDNA, known as "hot" regions, are situated between 303 and 315 nucleotides and between 16,184 and 16,193 nucleotides [6,13–15]. In addition, the D-loop of mtDNA contained multiple point mutations, microsatellite instability alterations, and significant deletions. These modifications may influence mtDNA replication and the transcription of mitochondrial genes [17]. The mitochondrial genome encodes thirteen essential subunits of the oxidative phosphorylation (OXPHOS) machinery in the inner mitochondrial membrane [14]. There are 13 mitochondrial genes that encode respiratory chain-related proteins, 22 that encode transfer RNA (tRNA), and the remaining 2 encode ribosomal RNA (rRNA)—12SrRNA and 16SrRNA [13]. The respiratory chain of the mitochondria has 87 polypeptides. Both the mitochondrial genome (mtDNA) and the nuclear genome encode the proteins that construct the inner mitochondrial membrane respiratory chain (nDNA). The respiratory chain proteins encoded by mitochondrial DNA include complex I—NADH proteins. Complex II, which regulates succinate dehydrogenase, is encoded exclusively by nuclear DNA [18]. The non-coding region of the D-loop is responsible for the control of mtDNA replication and transcription. The straightforward arrangement of mtDNA renders this genome more susceptible to the action of mutagenesis agents, such as those that affect the nuclear genome. Thus, the same cell can contain both normal copies of mitochondrial DNA and their mutants. This occurrence is referred to as heteroplasmia [19].

1.3. Diseases Related to mtDNA

Several studies have demonstrated a link between genetic alterations in mitochondrial DNA and human disorders, including coronary heart disease, hypertension, diabetes, endometriosis, and cancer [20–22]. The hunt for the reasons of the aging processes has also drawn the attention of numerous researchers on the effect of oxidative stress on mtDNA alterations [23,24]. Mitochondria are the site of cellular energy transformations, and in particular the site of formation and storage of high-energy compounds. Tissues highly dependent on mitochondrial energy production are the heart, skeletal muscle, central nervous system, and kidney. Therefore, the cause of disturbances in the functioning of these organs may be a decrease in the efficiency of mitochondrial respiration caused by mtDNA mutations. The so-called mitochondrial illnesses are caused by mutations in the mitochondrial DNA [25]. Mutations in the structure and function of mitochondria disturb the proper functioning of these organelles and deregulate the apoptotic process, which is the root cause of numerous human disorders [26].

2. Material and Methods

2.1. Study Design

The purpose of this study was to determine the types and frequency of changes in the sequence of mitochondrial DNA nucleotides in the HV1 and HV2 regions and in the D-loop region encoding the 12S rDNA in postmenopausal women with essential arterial hypertension and hormonal abnormalities.

2.2. Study Population

The tests were conducted on 100 women, 53 postmenopausal and 47 premenopausal, at the Department of Internal Diseases, Outpatients Clinic, and Department of Gynecology at The 1st Independent Public Teaching Hospital of Medical University of Lublin, Poland.

2.3. Study Variables

Among 75% of the women in the study group, arterial hypertension was detected. In each case, the following tests were conducted: 1/medical examination consisting of an interview and physical examination; 2/measurement of blood pressure twice after rest; 3/24 h blood pressure and heart rate monitoring; and 4/investigation of mtDNA polymorphism in the HV1 and HV2 regions and the 12S rDNA coding region. During two medical appointments, a medical examination was conducted, and a questionnaire was used to collect data from the interview and medical examination. Blood pressure was measured twice in the examined women each time after a 10 min rest, using the mean value of these measurements.

Women with severe organic systemic diseases, previously diagnosed neoplastic diseases, previously diagnosed mitochondrial diseases, severe degenerative diseases, previously diagnosed secondary hypertension, previously diagnosed ischemic heart disease, a history of a heart attack or stroke, cardiomyopathies, congenital and acquired heart defects, previously diagnosed peripheral vascular diseases, diabetes, thyrotoxicosis, and thymoma were excluded from research.

2.4. Methods of Examination Conducted in Study

The postmenopausal phase was determined based on the patient's medical history (menopausal symptoms such as hot flashes, increased sweating, and amenorrhea lasting over a year) and hormonal status (increase in FSH (follicle stimulating hormone) > 30 U/L in the blood serum).

Essential hypertension (AH) was diagnosed based on systolic blood pressure (RRs) 140 mmHg and/or diastolic blood pressure (RRr) 90 mmHg, as well as history (previously diagnosed and/or treated hypertension). Based on the systolic and diastolic blood pressure values, the European Society of Hypertension (ESC) distinguished arterial hypertension groups as optimal pressure, normal, high normal, arterial hypertension 1o, 2o, and 3o [27].

Every patient with arterial hypertension had outpatient 24 h monitoring of blood pressure and heart rate (ABPM). The hours beginning at 6 a.m. to 11 p.m. were taken as the waking and daytime hours, taking into account individual differences. Nighttime rest is 11 p.m. to 6 a.m. During the day, systolic and diastolic blood pressure were measured three times per hour, whereas at night, they were measured twice per hour. Systolic blood pressure (RRs) $\geq$ 135 mmHg during the day and diastolic blood pressure (RRr) $\geq$ 85 mmHg during the day were considered to be elevated, according to the recommendations of the European Society of Hypertension, and systolic blood pressure (RRs) $\geq$ 120 mmHg and diastolic pressure during the night were elevated (RRr) $\geq$ 70 mmHg.

The criteria for a sudden morning rise in blood pressure were increases in systolic and diastolic blood pressure of at least 10 mmHg. The increase is the difference between the mean nighttime measurements taken during sleep and the first two hours after awakening.

According to the magnitude of the decrease in systolic blood pressure, the following subgroups were distinguished among women with hypertension before and after menopause: 1. "dippers"—decrease in systolic blood pressure at night (RRs) compared to the day from 10 to 20%, 2. "non-dippers"—night systolic blood pressure (RRs) decrease in relation to the day to 10%, 3. "extreme dippers"—systolic blood pressure (RRs) drops by more than 20% between day and night, 4. "reverse dippers"—increase in systolic blood pressure (RRs) at night.

2.4.1. Isolation of mtDNA Polymorphism in the Regions of HV1, HV2, and 12S rDNA

Blood was collected for genetic testing under standard fasting conditions. Blood cells (lymphocytes) of the patients were isolated using the QIAamp DNA Midi Kit (Qiagen, Hilden, Germany) according to the manufacturer's isolation protocol [28]. The purity and concentration of DNA were analyzed spectrophotometrically (SynergyTM H1, BioTek, Santa Clara, CA, USA). The obtained DNA was suspended in EB buffer (10 mM TrisHCl pH 8.5) and stored at −20 degrees Celsius for future research.

2.4.2. Analysis of the mtDNA D-Loop Mutation

MtDNA's D-loop region was amplified with two PCR primer pairs. The primers had the following sequences: F4 5′ CACAGGTCTATCACCCTATTAACCA 3′ located at 4–28 bp, R599 5′ TTGAGGAGGTAAGCTACAT 3′ located at 599–581 bp, and F15974 5′ ACTCCACCATTAGCACCCAAA 3′ located at 15,974–15,994 bp; R16564 5′ TGATGTCTTATTTAAGGGGAACGT 3′ F4 and R16564 primers had previously been described [14]. In a 30 L reaction volume containing 1 PCR buffer, 1 M of each forward and reverse primer, 1.5 mM $MgCl_2$, 200 M of each dNTP, and 1 U of Taq DNA polymerase, PCR amplifications were performed (Fermentas, Waltham, MA, USA). The PCR conditions were as follows: pre-denaturation at 95 °C for 15 min, followed by 40 cycles at 95 °C for 20 s, 57.6 °C for 45 s, 72 °C for 45 s, and a final extension at 72 °C for 6 min (for the F4 and R599 pair of primers); and pre-denaturation at 95 °C for 5 min, followed by 30 cycles at 95 °C for 30 s. The electrophoresis of PCR products amplified from D-loop mtDNA was carried out on 1.5% agarose gels. Following purification with the QIAquick PCR Purification Kit (Qiagen, Hilden, Germany) according to the manufacturer's instructions, all PCR products were sequenced (in forward and reverse directions). The D-loop region's nucleotide sequence was determined by comparing sequences to the Cambridge reference sequence (rCRS, NC 012920) [29].

2.4.3. DNA Sequencing

The PCR-purified DNA samples were sequenced automatically. The Laboratory of Molecular Biology Techniques in Poznan, Poland, was tasked with completing this phase of research [28].

2.4.4. Computer Evaluation

Chromas—Pro software (version 1.31) and DNAStar (MegAlign, Madison, WI, USA) were used to interpret the chromatograms of the sequenced DNA samples. The BLAST Align two success program and the BioEdit program were used to compare DNA sequences from different samples in order to detect mutations (NCBI database). NC 012920 was the sequence number selected from the databases as the reference sequence [29].

2.5. Ethics

Research procedures were in line with ethical standards for human experimentation. They were in accordance with the opinion of the Bioethics Committee of the Medical University of Lublin (No. KE-0254/185/2006, 26 October 2006) as well as the Helsinki Declaration of 1975 and its 2000 amendment. Each of the examined persons gave written informed consent to participate in the experiment.

2.6. Statistical Analysis

Using the Kolmogorov–Smirnov test (allowing for the assessment of the normality of the distribution), it was determined whether individual analyses including linear variables required parametric tests (Student's *t*-test used in the comparisons of two independent groups if the assessed variables had a normal data distribution) or non-parametric tests (U-Mann–Whitney test used in the comparisons of 2 independent groups or the Spearman's rank correlation test used to assess the correlation between 2 variables if the assessed variables had a distribution other than normal). In comparisons of linear variables, the mean was used as the measure of concentration, and the standard deviation as the measure of dispersion. As a result, the correlation coefficient R was calculated when evaluating the correlation. Moreover, in the case of nonlinear data (classified), their analysis was conducted using the logistic regression method, which included the calculation of Wald 2, odds ratios (ORs), and corresponding 95% confidence intervals (95%CI). In all analyses, alpha (*p*-value) values less than 0.05 were considered statistically significant.

3. Results

3.1. Age and Anthropometric Information Regarding the Respondents

A group of 100 non-smoking and non-alcohol-using women before (47 women) and after menopause (53 women), mean age 51.1 ± 5.0 years, mean body weight 70.3 ± 14.5 kg, BMI (body mass index) (kg/m^2)- 27.2 ± 5.3, waist circumference (cm) 87.7 ± 13.7, and WHR waist/hip ratio 0.829 ± 0.061, was examined. The range of time since the last menstrual period was 0 to 7.9 years, with a mean of 4.5 to 7.9 years. No participant had ever utilized Hormone Replacement Therapy. The studied groups of pre- and postmenopausal women did not differ in terms of body weight, BMI, waist circumference, or WHR. A statistically significant difference existed between the age of the group of women studied before and after menopause. Women in the postmenopausal group were older than in the premenopausal group, and the difference was statistically significant ($p < 0.01$).

The average age of respondents with mtDNA polymorphism (before and after menopause) was 52.0 4.8 years and did not differ significantly from the average age of the other respondents (50.8 5.1 years; $p = 0.131$).

3.2. Analysis of the Sequences of the mtDNA HV1, HV2, and 12S RNA Regions

The nucleotide sequence of the most variable regions of the D-loop, HV1 and HV2, and the coding region of the 12S RNA of mtDNA were analyzed in total DNA isolated from the blood cells of 53 postmenopausal women and 47 premenopausal women who served as the reference group. A summary of the observed changes in the studied mtDNA regions in the entire group of women (in the pre- and postmenopausal period) is presented in Table 1.

In the group of 100 women (before and after the menopause), changes in the nucleotide sequence in the mtDNA segments studied were found in 23% of cases. The number of females and variations in the nucleotide sequence of mtDNA were as follows:

- With all mtDNA nucleotide sequence changes in the HV1 and HV2 regions and mtDNA 12S RNA coding sequence—23 women.
- With nucleotide sequence changes in the HV1 mtDNA region—14 women.
- With nucleotide sequence changes in the HV2 mtDNA region—11 women.
- With nucleotide sequence changes in the HV1 and HV2 regions of mtDNA—21 women.

- With changes in the coding sequence of nucleotides in the 12S RNA region of mtDNA—12 women.

Table 1. List of changes in mtDNA in the HV1, HV2, and 12S RNA regions in the entire study group of women and in the group of pre- and postmenopausal women.

mtDNA Region	Nucleotide Position in mtDNA	Sequence according to the MITOWEB Database *	Change	% Changes in mtDNA in the Entire Study Group	% Changes in mtDNA in the Premenopausal Study Group	% Changes in mtDNA in the Postmenopausal Study Group
MT-HV2	73 (-)	A	A-G	5 (5%)	0	5 (9.4%)
MT-OHR	127 (-)	T	T-C	1 (1%)	1 (2.1%)	0
MT-HV2	146 (-)	T	T-C	1 (1%)	0	1(1.9%)
MT-HV2	150 (-)	C	C-T	2 (2%)	0	2 (3.8%)
MT-OHR	152 (-)	T	T-C	2 (2%)	0	2 (3.8%)
MT- HV2	195 (-)	T	T-C	3 (3%)	0	3 (5.7%)
MT-OHR	199 (-)	T	T-C	1 (1%)	0	1(1.9%)
MT-OHR	204 (-)	T	T-C	1 (1%)	0	1(1.9%)
MT-OHR	207 (-)	G	G-A	1 (1%)	0	1 (1.9%)
MT-TFX	239	T	T-C	1 (1%)	0	1 (1.9%)
MT-TFX	243	A	A-G	1 (1%)	0	1 (1.9%)
MT-TFX	247	G	G-A	1 (1%)	0	1 (1.9%)
MT-OHR	250	T	T-C	1 (1%)	0	1 (1.9%)
MT-TFX	260	G	G-A	1 (1%)	0	1 (1.9%)
MT-OHR	263 (-)	A	A-G	9 (9%)	0	9 (17.0%)
MT-OHR	264 (-)	C	C-T	1 (1%)	0	1 (1.9%)
MT-OHR	266 (-)	T	T-G	1 (1%)	0	1 (1.9%)
MT-TFY	277	C	C-T	1 (1%)	1	0
MT-TFY	284	C	C-T	1 (1%)	1 (2.1%)	0
MT-TFY	295	C	C-T	1 (1%)	0	1 (1.9%)
MT-CBS2	310	C	C-T	3 (3%)	0	3 (5.7%)
MT-CBS2	311	C	C-T	2 (2%)	0	2 (3.8%)
MT-HPR	319	T	T-C	1 (1%)	0	1 (1.9%)
MT-OHR	338 (-)	C	C-T	1 (1%)	0	1 (1.9%)
MT-OHR	340 (-)	C	C-A	1 (1%)	0	1 (1.9%)
MT-CBS3	362	T	T-C	1 (1%)	0	1 (1.9%)
MT-HV3	480	T	T-C	1 (1%)	0	1 (1.9%)
MT-3H	385	A	A-G	1 (1%)	0	1 (1.9%)
MT-HV3	477 (-)	T	T-C	1 (1%)	0	1 (1.9%)
MT-HV3	489 (-)	T	T-C	1 (1%)	0	1 (1.9%)
MT-RNR1	709 (-)	G	G-A	1 (1%)	0	1 (1.9%)
MT-RNR1	750 (-)	A	A-G	10 (10%)	0	10 (18.9%)
MT-RNR1	812 (-)	A	A-G	1 (1%)	0	1 (1.9%)
MT-RNR1	930 (-)	G	G-A	2 (2%)	0	2 (3.8%)

Table 1. *Cont.*

mtDNA Region	Nucleotide Position in mtDNA	Sequence according to the MITOWEB Database *	Change	% Changes in mtDNA in the Entire Study Group	% Changes in mtDNA in the Premenopausal Study Group	% Changes in mtDNA in the Postmenopausal Study Group
MT-RNR1	961 (-)	T	T-G	1 (1%)	0	1 (1.9%)
MT-RNR1	1189	G	G-C	1 (1%)	0	1 (1.9%)
MT-RNR1	1438 (-)	A	A-G	10 (10%)	0	10 (18.9%)
MT-HV1	16,069 (-)	C	C-T	2 (2%)	0	2 (3.8%)
MT-7SDNA	16,093 (-)	T	T-C	1 (1%)	1 (2.1%)	0
MT-HV1	16,126 (-)	T	T-C	5 (5%)	1	4
MT-HV1	16,129 (-)	G	G-A	1 (1%)	0	1 (1.9%)
MT-HV1	16,140 (-)	T	T-C	1 (1%)	0	1 (1.9%)
MT-7SDNA	16,145 (-)	G	G-A	2 (2%)	1 (2.1%)	1 (1.9%)
MT-HV1	16,147 (-)	C	C-T	1 (1%)	1 (2.1%)	0
MT-HV1	16,174	C	C-T	1 (1%)		1 (1.9%)
MT-DLOOP	16,176 (-)	C	C-G	1 (1%)	1 (2.1%)	0
MT-HV1	16,189 (-)	T	T-C	1 (1%)	0	1 (1.9%)
MT-DLOOP	16,192 (-)	C	C-T	1 (1%)	0	1 (1.9%)
MT-HV1	16,222 (-)	C	C-T	1 (1%)	0	1 (1.9%)
MT-HV1	16,223 (-)	C	C-T	3 (3%)	1 (2.1%)	2
MT-DLOOP	16,224 (-)	T	T-C	1 (1%)	0	1 (1.9%)
MT-DLOOP	16,230 (-)	A	A-G	1 (1%)	1 (2.1%)	0
MT-DLOOP	16,256 (-)	C	C-T	1 (1%)	0	1 (1.9%)
MT-HV1	16,261 (-)	C	C-T	2 (2%)	0	2 (3.8%)
MT-DLOOP	16,263 (-)	T	T-C	1 (1%)	1 (2.1%)	0
MT-HV1	16,264 (-)	C	C-T	1 (1%)	0	1(1.9%)
MT-HV1	16,266 (-)	C	C-A	1 (1%)	0	1 (1.9%)
MT-DLOOP	16,270 (-)	C	C-T	3 (3%)	0	3 (5.7%)
MT-DLOOP	16,286 (-)	C	C-T	1 (1%)	1 (2.1%)	0
MT-HV1	16,288 (-)	T	T-C	1 (1%)	0	1 (1.9%)
MT-HV1	16,292 (-)	C	C-T	1 (1%)	0	1 (1.9%)
MT-HV1	16,294 (-)	C	C-T	2 (2%)	1 (2.1%)	1 (1.9%)
MT-HV1	16,296 (-)	C	C-T	2 (2%)	1 (2.1%)	1 (1.9%)
MT-DLOOP	16,298 (-)	T	T-C	1 (1%)	1 (2.1%)	0
MT-HV1	16,304 (-)	T	T-C	2 (2%)	1 (2.1%)	1 (1.9%)
MT-HV1	16,311 (-)	T	T-C	3 (3%)	0	3
MT- HPR	16,319	G	G-A	1 (1%)	0	1 (1.9%)
MT-HV1	16,362 (-)	T	T-C	2 (2%)	0	2
MT-DLOOP	16,390 (-)	G	G-A	1 (1%)	1 (2.1%)	0

Table 1. *Cont.*

mtDNA Region	Nucleotide Position in mtDNA	Sequence according to the MITOWEB Database *	Change	% Changes in mtDNA in the Entire Study Group	% Changes in mtDNA in the Premenopausal Study Group	% Changes in mtDNA in the Postmenopausal Study Group
MT-DLOOP	16,391 (-)	G	G-A	1 (1%)	0	1 (1.9%)
MT-DLOOP	16,497 (-)	A	A-G	1 (1%)	0	1 (1.9%)
MT-DLOOP	16,519 (-)	T	T-C	8 (8%)	4 (8.5%)	4 (7.6%)
MT-DLOOP	16,526 (-)	G	G-A	1 (1%)	0	1 (1.9%)

* According to the MITOWEB database, www.mitomap.org (accessed 31 January 2023) [28]: (-), non-coding nucleotide MT-RNR1 ribosomal RNA (12S RNA mtDNA); MT-HV1, hypervariable segment 1 (from nucleotide 16,024 to 16,365); MT-HV2, hypervariable segment 2 (from nucleotide 73 to 340); MT-HV3, hypervariable segment 3; MT-OHR, H-strand origin; MT-CBS2, conserved sequence block 2 (conserved sequence box); MT-CBS3, conserved sequence block 3 (conserved sequence box); MT-TFX, mtTF1 binding site; MT-TFY, mtTF1 binding site; MT-HPR, replication primer; MT-7SDNA-7SDNA; MT-3H, mt3 H-strand control element.

The number of observed mtDNA changes in individual cases ranged from 1 to 18. They were present in 91.3% of the hypervariable regions (HV1 and HV2), and more frequently in the HV1 segment (60.9%) than the HV2 segment (47.5%). The number of observed changes in individual cases ranged from one to nine.

Changes were present in 43.5% of the 12S RNA coding region, where from two to five changes were observed. Changes in the mtDNA nucleotide sequence affected the HV1 segment in 60.9% of cases, the HV2 segment in 47.8% of cases, and the number of changes observed in individual cases ranged from one to nine. In 47.8% of cases with two to five lesions, mtDNA changes occurred in the 12S RNA coding sequence.

Changes in the Nucleotide Sequence of the HV1, HV2, and 12S RNA Regions of mtDNA are Presented in Table 2.

3.3. *Homoplasmia/Heteroplasmia of mtDNA in the Study Group with Changes in the Mitochondrial Genome in the HV1 and HV2 mtDNA Regions*

Most of the identified changes in the nucleotide sequence are homoplasmic (81.8% of respondents with changes in the HV1 region, 90.1% in the HV2 region, and 100% with changes in the region encoding the 12S RNA mtDNA). Heteroplasmic changes concerned the following nucleotides in the HV1 region: 16093TC, 16230AG, and 16286CT occurred in 18.2% of the subjects with changes in the HV1 region. In subjects with the 239TC nucleotide the changes in the HV2 region were detected in 9.9% cases.

3.4. *Menopause*

The frequency of nucleotide sequence changes in the mitochondrial genome of the studied postmenopausal women (34.0%) compared to the premenopausal period (10.6%) was significantly higher ($p = 0.016$). Both changes in the HV2 region and in the 12S RNA coding sequence occurred only in the studied postmenopausal women and were not observed in the studied group of premenopausal women. The frequency of nucleotide sequence changes in both HV1 and HV2 hypervariable segments in postmenopausal women was higher compared to the premenopausal period, and the difference was statistically significant ($p = 0.011$).

However, the incidence of mtDNA changes among the examined postmenopausal women in the HV1 segment only did not differ significantly in comparison to the group of premenopausal women. A comparison of the frequency of nucleotide sequence changes in different mtDNA segments in pre- and postmenopausal women is presented in Table 3.

Table 2. Distribution of nucleotide changes in HV1, HV2, and 12S RNA regions of mtDNA of all patients.

Location	Others	Modifications	Cases (%)
HV1		16519TC	64.2
		16126TC	35.7
		16311TC, 16223CT, and 16270CT	21.4
		16069CT, 16145GA, 16261CT, 16294CT, 16296CT, 16304TC, and 16362TC	14.3
		16093TC, 16129GA, 16140TC, 16147CT, 16174CT, 16176CG, 16189TC, 16192CT, 16222CT, 16224TC, 16230AG, 16256CT, 16263TC, 16264CT, 16266CA, 16286CT, 16288TC 16292CGA, 16319GA, 16291GA, 16292TCGA, 16319GA, 16319GA, and 16319GA	7.1
HV2		263AG	81.8
		73AG	45.5
		195TC	27.3
		150CT, 152TC	18.2
	Transcription factor binding site	239TC, 243AG, 247GA, 250TC, 260GA, 277CT, 284CT, and 295CT	36.4
	Coding region—CBS3	310CT	27.3
	Coding region—CBS3	311CT	18.2
12S RNA		1438AG, 750AG	90
		930GA	20
		709GA, 812AG, 961TG, and 1189GC	10
	Section MT3H	385AG	1
	Section HV3	477TC	1
	Section HV3	489TC	1
	Section HV3	480TC	1

Table 3. Comparison of the frequency of nucleotide sequence changes in different mtDNA segments in the studied groups of pre- and postmenopausal women.

Changes	Premenopausal Women	Postmenopausal Women	X^2 Walda	Odds Ratio	Range	*p*-Value
	47 (47%)	53 (53%)				
mtDNA	5 (10.6%)	18 (34.0%)	6.0	3.9	1.29–11.8	0.016
HV1	5 (10.6%)	9 (17.0%)	0.55	1.56	0.48–5.1	0.457
HV2	0 (0%)	11 (20.8%)	n/a			
HV1+HV2	5 (10.6%)	16 (30.2%)	6.4	4.6	1.4–15.1	0.011
12S DRNA	0 (0%)	12 (22.6%)	n/a			

Modifications in the nucleotide sequence in mtDNA occurred in women with hypertension (pre- and postmenopausal) in 25.3% of the subjects. Changes in the nucleotide sequence in mtDNA in postmenopausal women with arterial hypertension occurred in 37.5% of the respondents and in 11.5% of the premenopausal women. The difference was statistically significant ($p = 0.030$).

Table 4 presents a comparison of the frequency of mtDNA nucleotide sequence changes in the hypervariable sections of HV1 and HV2 and the coding sequence of 12S RNA with arterial hypertension in the premenopausal group and the postmenopausal group. The frequencies of nucleotide sequence changes in the HV1, HV2, and 12S rDNA mtDNA regions in pre- and postmenopausal hypertension are presented (37.5% vs. 11.5%, $p = 0.03$).

Table 4. The frequency of nucleotide sequence changes in various mtDNA regions in the group of women with arterial hypertension depending on the menopausal status.

	Premenopausal Group	Postmenopausal Group	X^2 Walda	Odds Ratio	Range	p-Value
Number of cases	35 (74.5%)	40 (75.5%)				
Changes HV1, HV2, 12S rDNA	4 (11.5%)	15 (37.5%)	4.7	3.9	1.1–13.8	0.030
HV1	4 (11.5%)	10 (25%)	0.39	1.5	0.39–5.9	0.529
HV2	0 (0%)	10 (25%)	n/a			
HV1 + HV2	4 (11.5%)	14 (35%)	5.9	5.4	1.4–21.6	0.015
12S rDNA	0 (0%)	10 (25%)	n/a			

In subjects with premenopausal hypertension, no changes in mtDNA nucleotide sequence in the HV2 and 12S RNA segment were observed; hence, the influence of menopausal status on the incidence of these changes cannot be statistically expressed.

3.5. Parameters of Daily RR Monitoring in Patients with Arterial Hypertension Depending on Changes in mtDNA Nucleotide Sequence

Changes in the HV1 and HV2 regions of mtDNA were accompanied by a modification of the parameters of the monitored RR. Statistically significantly higher maximum systolic RR and heart rate/min were observed, as well as a higher frequency of increased values of systolic RR during the day in the subjects (before and after menopause) in the group with nucleotide sequence changes in the HV1 and HV2 segments compared to the group without these changes. Parameters of daily RR monitoring in the subjects (before and after menopause) in the group with changes in the nucleotide sequence in the HV1 and HV2 regions and in the group without these changes are presented in Figures 1 and 2.

3.6. Nucleotide Sequence Changes in HV1 and RR Monitoring

Alterations in the nucleotide sequence in the HV1 segment were associated with an increase in maximum daytime systolic blood pressure. The mean maximum systolic RR in the patients (before and after menopause) in the group with nucleotide sequence changes in the HV1 hypervariable region was statistically significantly higher compared to the group without these changes. The remaining parameters of the daily RR monitoring did not differ significantly in the studied women (before and after the menopause) between the group with changes in the nucleotide sequence in the HV1 segment as compared to the group without changes. A comparison of these parameters is presented in Figure 3.

3.7. Nucleotide Sequence Changes in HV2 and RR Monitoring

Modifications in the nucleotide sequence in the HV2 mtDNA region were accompanied by slightly higher mean values of the maximum systolic RR both during the day and night, as well as significantly higher heart rate/min during the day. The comparison of RR monitoring parameters in the subjects (pre- and postmenopausal) in the group with changes in the nucleotide sequence in the HV2 hypervariable region to the group without changes is presented in Figure 4.

3.8. Nucleotide Coding Sequence Changes in 12S RNA and RR Monitoring

Changes in the nucleotide sequence in the 12S RNA coding region were associated with the modification of the parameters of the monitored RR in their presence, but only in a way close to statistical significance. Maximum daytime and nighttime systolic RR and daytime heart rate were slightly higher in the group of subjects with nucleotide sequence changes in the coding region of the 12S RNA compared to the corresponding values in the group without these changes. The differences in each case were close to statistical significance. The other parameters of the monitored pressure showed no differences between these groups. These data are presented in Figure 5.

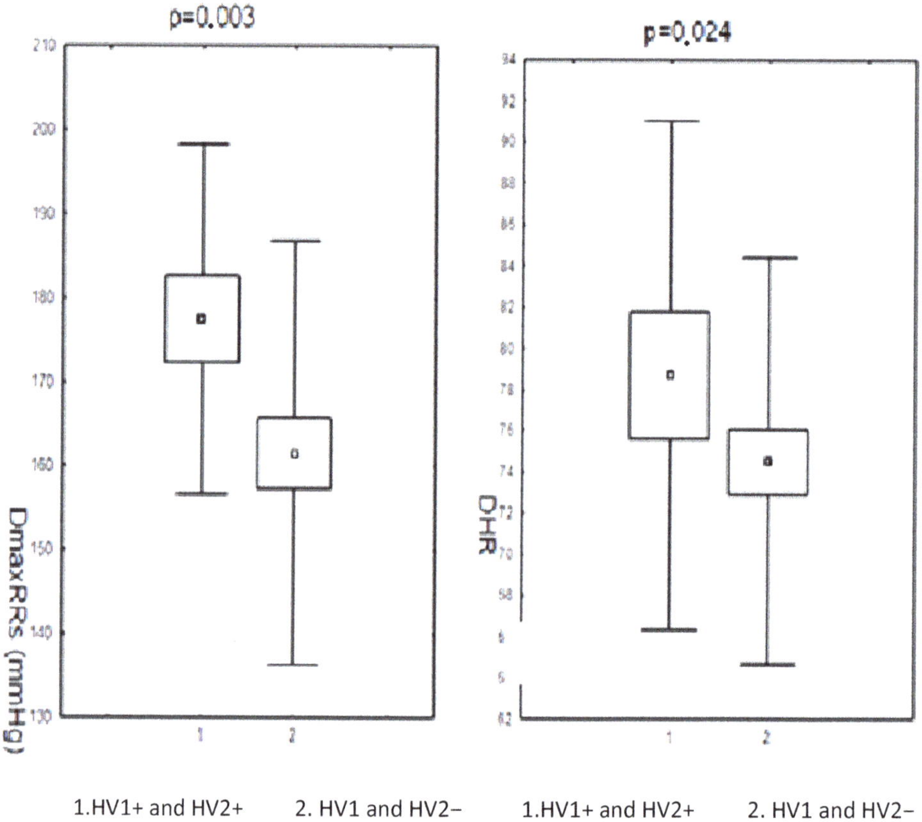

Figure 1. Results of 24 h measurements of systolic blood pressure during the day and heart rate in patients (pre- and postmenopausal) with arterial hypertension depending on changes in the nucleotide sequence in the HV1 and HV2 segment. DmaxRR—daytime maximum blood pressure; DHR—daily heart rate; HV1 and HV2+—positive for HV1 and HV2 changes; HV1 and HV2−—negative for HV1 and HV2 changes.

3.9. MtDNA Nucleotide Sequence Changes and Morning Rises in Blood Pressure

Nucleotide sequence changes in the HV1 and HV2 regions were associated with a slightly more frequent occurrence of morning increases in blood pressure, but without statistical significance. Both changes in the HV1 and HV2 regions separately and in the region of the 12S RNA coding sequence were not associated with more frequent morning increases in RR.

3.10. Nocturnal Drops in Blood Pressure and Changes in mtDNA Nucleotide Sequence

The percentage of reduction in systolic blood pressure at night in the premenopausal group with mtDNA nucleotide sequence changes was 15.7% and in the postmenopausal group with mtDNA changes was 11.1%, and the difference was not statistically significant, $p = 0.180$.

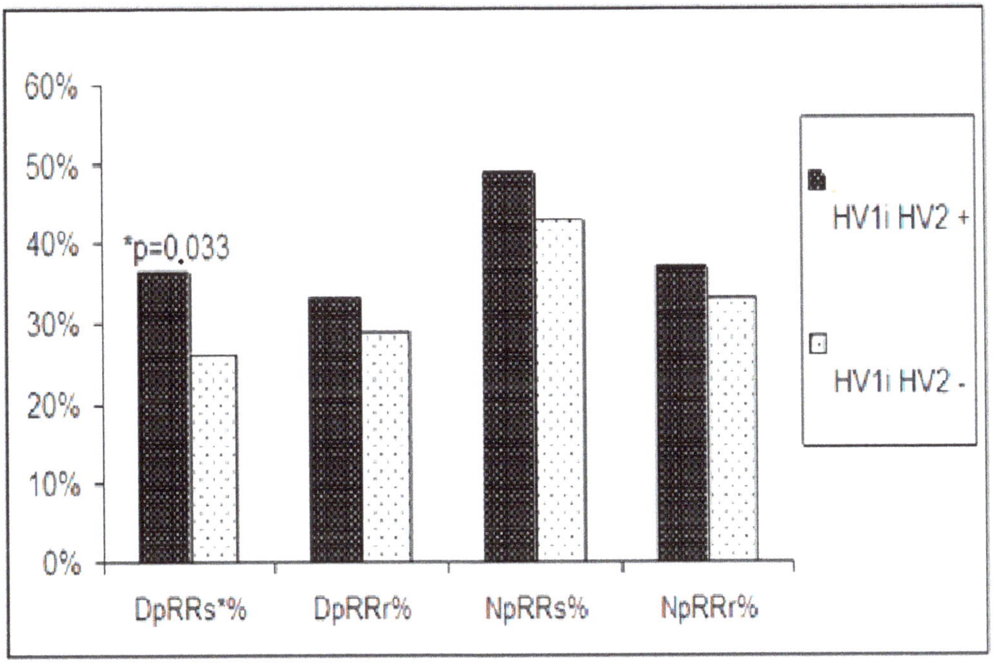

Figure 2. Comparison of the incidence of elevated blood pressure measurements obtained during 24 h blood pressure monitoring in pre- and postmenopausal women with hypertension. DpRRs%-percentage of increased systolic blood pressure values during the day; DpRRr%-percentage of increased diastolic blood pressure values during the day; NpRRs%-percentage of elevated systolic blood pressure values at night; NpRRr%-percentage of elevated diastolic blood pressure values at night. * denotes p value.

The frequency of the subgroups of hypertension—dippers, extreme dippers, reverse dippers, and non-dippers—was not dependent on changes in the nucleotide sequence in mtDNA. The difference in the incidence of these subgroups of hypertension in the subjects (pre- and postmenopausal) in the group with mtDNA nucleotide sequence changes compared to the group without these changes was statistically insignificant ($p = 0.116$). These data are presented in Table 5.

3.11. Summary

- Changes in the examined mtDNA segments occurred in 23% of women, more often after than before menopause, and in some areas they occurred only after menopause (12S rDNA, HV2). Most often they concerned the HV1 segment, but a slightly smaller percentage of patients showed changes in the HV2 segment and the 12S RNA coding sequence.
- Changes in mtDNA, regardless of localization, were associated with the course of arterial hypertension, greater and more frequent increases in systolic blood pressure, morning increases in blood pressure, and higher heart rate, suggesting adrenergic stimulation in these subjects.

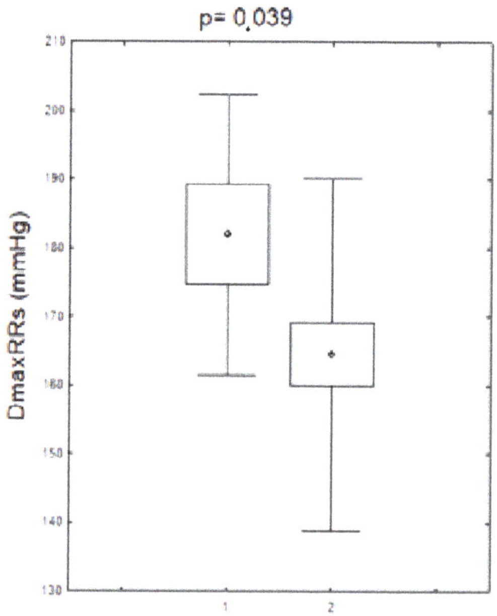

Figure 3. Maximum systolic blood pressure values during the day in patients (pre- and postmenopausal) with arterial hypertension with the changes in the HV1 regions. DDmaxRRs-daily maximum systolic blood pressure, HV1+,-positive for HV1 changes, HV1−,-negative for HV1 changes.

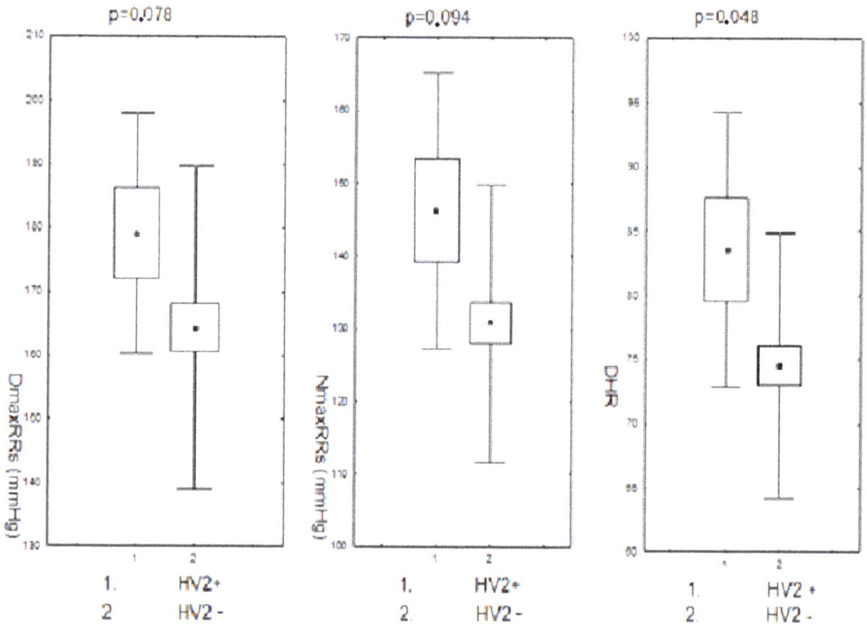

Figure 4. Maximum systolic blood pressure during the day and night and heart rate/min during the day in pre- and postmenopausal women with hypertension with changes in the HV2 regions. DDmaxRRs-daily maximum systolic blood pressure; NmaxRRs-nighttime maximum systolic blood pressure; DHR-daily heart rate; HV2+,-positive for HV2 changes; HV2−,-negative for HV2 changes.

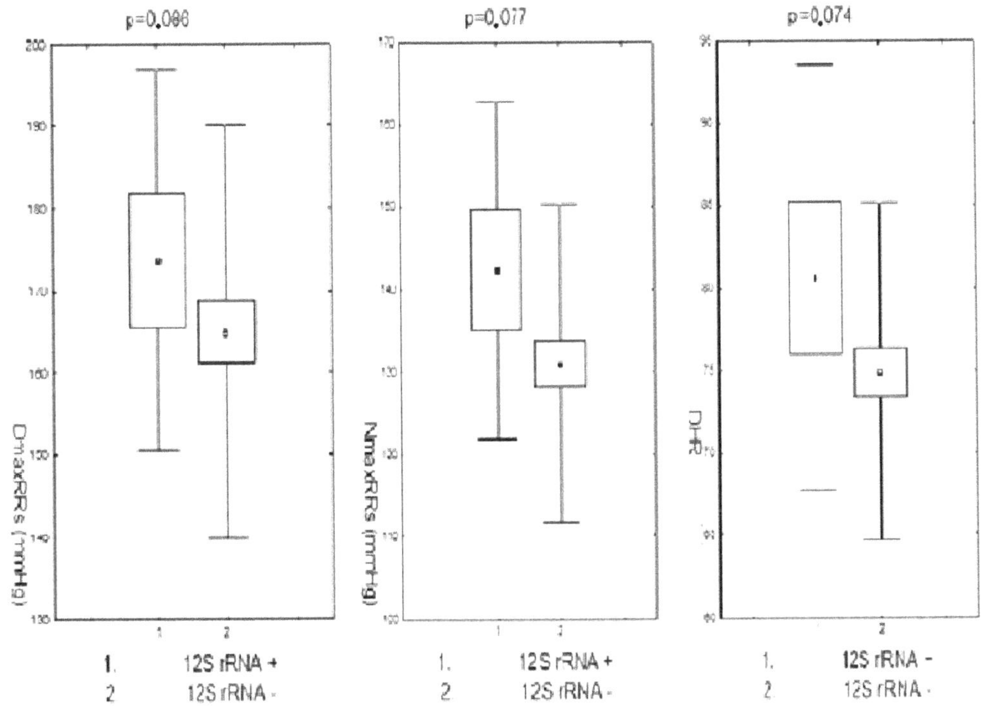

Figure 5. Maximum systolic blood pressure during the day and night and heart rate during the day in pre- and postmenopausal patients with arterial hypertension and in the region of the 12S RNA coding sequence. DDmaxRRs-daily maximum systolic blood pressure; NmaxRRs-nighttime maximum systolic blood pressure; DHR-daily heart rate; 12SrRNA+,-positive for 12SrRNA changes; 12SrRNA−,-negative for 12SrRNA changes.

Table 5. The incidence of hypertension subgroups (dippers, extreme dippers, reverse dippers, and non-dippers) depending on the presence of nucleotide sequence changes in mtDNA.

	All Changes +	All Changes −	*p*-Value
AH (number)	18	57	
"dippers"	52.9%	34.2%	0.166
"non-dippers"	29.4%	53.7%	
"extreme dippers"	5.8%	7.3%	
"reverse dippers"	11.8%	4.9%	

4. Discussion

4.1. Rationale of the Study

The demographic structure of European societies has changed dramatically over the past decades. Data from 2020 show that 20.6% of people in European countries are over 65 [30]. The population aged 80 years or above in the EU's population is projected to have a 2.5-fold increase between 2020 and 2100, from 5.9% to 14.6. This fact changes the tasks of medical care in European societies. Thus, women live nearly 10 years longer than men. The process of individual aging is easier to define in women due to the presence of menopause, which takes a woman from the period of full life and reproductive activity to the postmenopausal period leading to old age. Degenerative diseases, cardiovascular diseases, metabolic diseases, and neoplastic diseases occurring with the aging process determine the quality of life later in life. They have their genesis in molecular changes, in which mitochondrial dysfunctions play a non-negligible role, which may be related to the growth and accumulation of mutations within the mitochondrial genome [31].

4.2. mtDNA Polymorphism and Its Relation to Diseases and Aging

Single-nucleotide polymorphism studies allowed to determine genotypes responsible for a specific disease in monogenic diseases, and recently also genotypes with a high risk of multigene diseases [32,33]. One of the possible consequences of an mtDNA mutation—monogenic diseases—is rare. For example, various mtDNA mutations may be responsible for the monogenic mitochondrial disease—Leber's hereditary optic neuropathy (LHON)—and 90% of patients have one of them: 11778G/A; 3460G/A; and 14484T/C. These mutations in the population are found with a frequency of 1/300 [34]. Changes in the nucleotide sequence in mtDNA are easy, easier than in the nuclear genome, which is associated with exposure of the mitochondrial genome to contact with continuously produced reactive oxygen species, as well as reduced mtDNA repair possibilities [35,36]. More frequent occurrence of mtDNA mutations in older age groups of patients was observed by Michikawa et al. [37]. Changes in the mtDNA nucleotide sequence occurred in the majority (in 57% of the studied patients) of the studied patients over 65 years of age, which, however, were not observed in the groups of younger patients. With age, the progressive increase in mtDNA mutations as a result of reaction to reactive oxygen species is secondary to lipid oxidation and the modification of mitochondrial proteins in the cell's respiratory chain [38,39]. MtDNA mutations change the structure of the respiratory chain polypeptides encoded in the mitochondrial genome, reducing mitochondrial metabolic activity and the formation of high-energy compounds [40]. Respiratory chain enzymes encoded by altered mtDNAs disrupt electron transport, increase electron leakage from the respiratory chain, and increase the amount of free oxygen radicals produced, further damaging the mitochondria and creating a vicious circle effect. This mechanism leads to the deterioration of the functioning of organs and tissues during the aging process. Modification of apoptosis signaling secondary to mitochondrial damage has been observed in in vivo and in vitro studies. This thesis is confirmed by the results of studies by Wei et al. on skin fibroblasts [41]. The above-mentioned researchers observed greater disturbances in fibroblast bioenergetics in the elderly compared to younger people, which was assessed on the basis of a higher concentration of hydrogen peroxide, a high level of superoxide dismutase activity, and a decrease in the activity of cytochrome c oxidase, as well as the oxygen consumption rate in the older age group. At the same time, a decrease in pyruvate dehydrogenase (PDH) expression and an increase in lactate dehydrogenase kinase were observed.

4.3. Study Subjects and Comparison of Results with Previous Studies

Despite the relationships of mtDNA polymorphism with age repeatedly described in the scientific literature, our studies did not show significant differences in age between the groups of women studied with changes in nucleotide sequences in the D-loop and without mtDNA changes. MtDNA changes with age, hence, we studied women over 40 (between 40–60 years old). The restricted age range of the research group may have prevented age disparities between women with mtDNA nucleotide sequence alterations and those without. Disturbances in the physiological functions of mitochondria may depend not only on the direct effect of the mutation on the respiratory chain, but may also occur secondary to the existing multigene disease and dysfunction of the mitochondrial respiratory chain in its course. However, it should be emphasized that certain mtDNA mutations may be beneficial. There are publications regarding changes in nucleotide sequences in mtDNA accompanying longevity. Studies by Kokaze et al. found that the mtDNA 5178 C/A polymorphism, which is associated with longevity, may prevent the onset of diabetes [42]. It has been shown that this genotype reduces the number of mtDNA mutations in oocytes, as well as the rate of mtDNA mutation formation and their accumulation in somatic cells in Japanese centenarians. The mtDNA 5178 C/A polymorphism not only prevents diabetes but is probably responsible for inhibiting the development of myocardial infarction [43]. Zhang et al., in the Italian population, studied the frequency of the C150T mutation located near the sequences responsible for mtDNA heavy strand synthesis. Its occurrence was more frequent in older age groups [44]. It appeared in approximately 17% of people (33/52) aged 99–106, while in younger people (aged 18–98) only in 3.4% (3/117).

Howell et al. and others found that mutations associated with multigenetic illnesses commonly occur in the D-loop region, a 1122 bp non-coding stretch of mtDNA containing two hypervariable regions, HV1 and HV2 [45,46]. This area has higher mtDNA polymorphism than others. Del Bo et al. found more mutations in the HV1 and HV2 hypervariable regions of the D-loop than other mtDNA segments in aged people [47]. Mutations in D-loop mtDNA nucleotide sequences, which occur often, disrupt mitochondrial genome replication and transcription. A single-nucleotide polymorphism in the D-loop and 12S RNA coding sequence of mtDNA was detected in 23% of our respondents. Like the aforementioned authors, we found more frequent changes in the hypervariable segments HV1 and HV2 of the D-loop, which occurred in 21.0% of respondents, somewhat more often in the HV1 segment (14.0% of respondents) than in HV2. In the HV1 area, 85.7% of mutations were homoplasmic and non-coding, and just one patient implicated nucleotide 16319, the beginning site for mtDNA synthesis and light strand engaged in replication. Nucleotide sequence alterations in the HV2 region were homoplasmic in 90.1% of instances, connected to the transcription factor binding site in CBS3 (conserved block) in 36%, and occurred in nearly 30% of responses. The 12S rDNA region has 10% non-coding nucleotides, 90% 1438AG and 750AG, and 20% 930GA. Rydzanicz et al. found polymorphisms in the 12S rDNA region (G709A, G750A, G930A, T1243C, T1420C, and G1438A) at a frequency greater than 1% [48]. This study found two mtDNA polymorphisms in the HV2 hypervariable section of the mitochondrial genome that have not been previously reported. A postmenopausal woman with arterial hypertension and metabolic syndrome had a polymorphism. The non-coding nucleotide 340C/A in the H strand origin region between the DNA replication primer and the CBS3 block was changed. The second nucleotide sequence change included the non-coding nucleotide 362T/C and the conserved CBS3 block. Our postmenopausal control patient showed another polymorphism. It was in the mtDNA 12S RNA coding sequence and associated with the non-coding nucleotide 812A/C. Most of the other alterations in the investigated population include mutations associated with multigene illnesses, coronary artery disease, hypertension, diabetes, and neoplastic diseases, according to the literature [26,49,50]. In multigene diseases, the disease process in such cases is not caused by a single change in nucleotide sequences in mtDNA, but by changes in many genes. The presence of mtDNA polymorphisms is not a prerequisite for clinical symptoms of the disease, and changes in the mitochondrial genome occur only in some patients with clinical symptoms of the disease. Homoplastic mutations, which do not always translate into the phenotype of clinical disease symptoms, are often diagnosed at random. This fact is explained by many authors by the direct influence on the mitochondrial genome of the nuclear genome and the influence of epigenetic factors, while the disclosure of heterozygous mutations is conditioned by the proportion of mutated and normal mtDNA [51,52]. Most polymorphisms occur as a variant of the genotype not associated with the occurrence of a given disease, and changes in nucleotide sequences are often located only in the vicinity of genes responsible for a given disease entity. As a result of changes in mtDNA, the same mutation may cause various sets of clinical symptoms or be asymptomatic. In summary, mitochondrial mutations may cause phenotypic effects that are difficult to predict and may occur as pathogenic or only potentially pathogenic mutations.

The study found that alterations in mtDNA in HV1, HV2, and 12S rDNA may impact arterial hypertension by increasing blood pressure day and night and heart rate, suggesting an increased adrenergic system tone in these people. The HV2 segment (239TC, 243AG, 247GA, 250TC, 260GA, 277CT, and 284CT) alterations mostly affected transcription factor binding sites and non-coding nucleotides in the 12S RNA and HV1 coding regions. According to Pejovic et al., the nucleotide sequences in the hypervariable D-loop regions that replicate mtDNA and the degree of transcription factor binding can alter mtDNA synthesis and cell number [53]. The examined women's HV2 region alterations, which impact mtDNA synthesis and transcription factor binding, may affect blood pressure. Several studies link hypertension to mitochondrial metabolism and free oxygen radicals [49,54]. On the other hand, the authors of experimental studies describe various forms of damage to the mitochondrial respiratory chain, leading to an increase in the production of reactive oxygen species that affect the course of hypertension. The source of reactive oxygen species in blood vessels are vascular endothelial cells, fibroblasts, and vascular smooth muscle, in which NAD (P) H or NADH oxidase (nicotinamide adenine dinucleotide in reduced form) catalyzing the reduction of oxygen causes the formation of O2 - and large amounts of other free radical oxygen. NAD (P) H oxidase activation occurs under the influence of TNF-α, angiotensin, and nitric oxide synthase. Hydrogen peroxide is a vasoactive compound with vasoconstrictor properties. According to Rubanyi et al., peroxygen hydrogen chloride in reaction with nitric oxide can transform into peroxynitrite anion (ONOO–), which reduces the availability of nitric oxide and thus contributes to the development of hypertension [55]. According to Pryor et al., hydrogen peroxide directly affects the opening of potassium and calcium channels, and therefore is also responsible for vasodilation. In turn, nitric oxide synthase is a source of not only NO, but also O_2, which reduces the availability of NO [56]. According to the authors cited above, the balance between NO and O_2, is essential for the damage to the vessel wall, the state of vascular tone, and the development of arterial hypertension. The production of large amounts of free oxygen radicals activates the tyrosine phosphatase and tyrosine kinase pathways, influences the expression of transcription factors and mitogen-activated protein kinases, and changes the activity of ion channels. ROS directly increases the concentration of calcium ions in the cell, leading to vessel wall dysfunction and remodeling. The changes in mtDNA observed in the group of women we have studied, accompanying higher blood pressure values, are probably the result of damage to the mitochondria and the formation of ROS. Many of the available publications on mitochondrial mutations in studied patients with maternal hypertension refer to Asian populations [57–61]. Various degrees of arterial hypertension recognized in the presence of mutations were observed: mutation 4435A > G, with a 30% reduction in mitochondrial metabolism and mitochondrial tRNA transcription (Met); mutation 4263A > G, located at the site of transcription for isoleucine (5′ end of tRNA (Ile)), which decreased the efficiency of the tRNA replication process by about 46%; the 4401A > G nucleotide mutation located directly at the 5′ end of the tRNA (Met) and tRNA (Gln), with a reduction in the mitochondrial translation index and a reduction in the mitochondrial respiratory efficiency index; and mutation T3308C on the dehydrogenase subunit (ND1), in which the translation initiating amino acid-methionine has been replaced with tyronine in ND1, with the alteration of RNA precursor strand processing or destabilization of ND1-mtRNA dehydrogenase.

The results of this study and other investigations suggest that alterations in the mtDNA nucleotide sequence may cause arterial hypertension. A shortage of postmenopausal sex hormones may damage the mitochondrial respiratory chain, causing mtDNA alterations and hypertension as a multigene illness. The literature shows multigene alterations in mtDNA coding and non-coding nucleotides in arterial hypertension, comparable to our findings [62]. The function of mtDNA D-loop hypervariable regions in arterial hypertension was examined by Liu et al. Changes in the HV2 area 152T-> C, 182C-> T, and 247G-> A and HV1 segment 16187C-> T, 16189T-> C, 16264C-> T, 16270C-> T, and 16311T-> C predispose to essential hypertension. According to these authors, the development of hypertension does not correlate to the severity of the mutation's influence on the illness's clinical picture, and the environment and nuclear gene modifiers in these individuals also modify the mutation's effect on the disease. In a Japanese population investigation on the association between mtDNA alterations and arterial hypertension, Soji et al. found that the mtDNA genotype 16223TC is more prevalent in hypertensive patients than in those without hypertension and is associated with higher hypertension risk [63]. They found no connection with other genotypes, including C16362T. As in this study, studies on the mitochondrial genome generally focused on single or many gene coding or non-coding agents and their link with disease entities, such as hypertension.

4.4. Strength and Limitations of the Study

One of the limitations of our research is that it involved women from 40 to 60 years of age, who could be expected to have changes in mtDNA with age. Another issue perhaps would be the small age range of the study group, which meant that the differences in the age of the studied women with changes in mtDNA nucleotide sequences compared to the patients without changes did not occur.

The investigators did not investigate other factors leading to hypertension, such as nutrition, which is a drawback of the study. Obesity can induce hypertension and therefore have an impact on changes in the mitochondrial genome sequence.

Our discovery may have clinical relevance in that Hormone Replacement Therapy may have a protective effect on mtDNA mutation. Several experimental medicines have already reached the clinical phase with extremely promising findings, yet the likelihood of enrolling patients in clinical trials is limited.

5. Conclusions

Changes in the HV1 and HV2 segments of mitochondrial DNA are accompanied by a more severe course of arterial hypertension with symptoms of adrenergic stimulation (higher maximum systolic pressure during the day and night, more frequent increases in systolic pressure, more frequent morning increases in blood pressure, and higher average heart rate).

The course of arterial hypertension in the mtDNA polymorphism group was more severe than in the patients without these changes, and at the same time there were symptoms of increased tension of the adrenergic system (slightly higher maximum systolic RR during the day and night and higher heart rate during the day).

In the HV2 hypervariable segment the mtDNA changes not yet described in the literature were detected: in the non-coding nucleotide 340 C/A (in the heavy strand H region) and in the non-coding nucleotide 362 T/C (in the region including the conservative block CBS3) in a postmenopausal woman with hypertension and metabolic syndrome and in the non-coding nucleotide 812 (AC) (region 12S RNA) in a postmenopausal control patient.

Author Contributions: W.K.—data curation, formal analysis, investigation, equal writing. A.S.—formal analysis, software, visualization, equal writing. A.W.—concept, methodology, supervision, writing. A.G.-J.—investigation, methodology, resources, writing. J.M. (Jerzy Mosiewicz)—supervision, resources. J.M. (Jolanta Mieczkowska)—concept, data collection, funding, writing. All authors have read and agreed to the published version of the manuscript.

Funding: Medical University of Lublin, Poland, research no. 159/08.

Institutional Review Board Statement: The study was approved by the Bioethics Committee of the Medical University of Lublin (no. KE-0254/185/2006) and with the Helsinki Declaration of 1975 and the amendment from 2000. Each of the examined persons gave written informed consent to participate in the experiment.

Informed Consent Statement: Informed consent was obtained from all subjects involved in the study. Written informed consent has been obtained from the patient(s) to publish this paper.

Data Availability Statement: The datasets used and/or analyzed during the current study are available from the corresponding author on reasonable request. All of the mentioned genetic polymorphisms in our manuscript are already deposited in dbSNP at https://www.ncbi.nlm.nih.gov/snp/ (accessed on 31 January 2023). The reference sequence selected from the databases was the sequence number NC_012920.

Conflicts of Interest: The authors declare no conflict of interest.

Abbreviations

AH	arterial hypertension
Bp	base pair
HV1	hypervariable region 1
HV2	hypervariable region 2
mtDNA	mitochondrial genome
nDNA	nucleotide DNA
Nt	nucleotide
RR	blood pressure

References

1. Anderson, S.; Bankier, A.T.; Barrell, B.G.; de Bruijn, M.H.; Coulson, A.R.; Drouin, J.; Eperon, I.C.; Nierlich, D.P.; Roe, B.A.; Sanger, F.; et al. Sequence and organization of the human mitochondrial genome. *Nature* **1981**, *290*, 457–465. [CrossRef] [PubMed]
2. Wallace, D.C.; Zheng, X.X.; Lott, M.T.; Shoffner, J.M.; Hodge, J.A.; Kelley, R.I.; Epstein, C.M.; Hopkins, L.C. Familial mitochondrial encephalomyopathy (MERRF): Genetic, pathophysiological, andbiochemical characterization of a mitochondrial DNA disease. *Cell* **1988**, *55*, 601. [CrossRef] [PubMed]
3. Bartnik, E.; Lorenc, A.; Mroczek, K. Human mitochondria in health, disease, ageing and cancer. *J. Appl. Genet.* **2001**, *42*, 65–71. [PubMed]
4. Ladoukakis, E.D.; Zouros, E. Evolution and inheritance of animal mitochondrial DNA: Rules and exceptions. *J. Biol. Res.-Thessaloniki* **2017**, *24*, 1–7. [CrossRef]
5. Shuster, R.C.; Rubenstein, A.J.; Wallace, D.C. Mitochondrial DNA in anucleate human blood cells. *Biochem. Biophys. Res. Commun.* **1988**, *155*, 1360–1365. [CrossRef]
6. Taanman, J.W. The mitochondrial genome: Structure, transcription, translation and replication. *Biochim. Biophys. Acta—Bioenerg.* **1999**, *1410*, 103–123. [CrossRef]
7. Cannino, G.; Di Liegro, C.M.; Rinaldi, A.M. Nuclear-mitochondrial interaction. *Mitochondrion* **2007**, *7*, 359–366. [CrossRef]
8. Endo, T.; Yamano, K. Multiple pathways for mitochondrial protein traffic. *Biol. Chem.* **2009**, *390*, 723–730. [CrossRef]
9. Herrmann, J.M.; Longen, S.; Weckbecker, D.; Depuydt, M. Biogenesis of mitochondrial proteins. *Adv. Exp. Med. Biol.* **2012**, *748*, 41–64.
10. Li, H.; Liu, D.; Lu, J.; Bai, Y. Physiology and pathophysiology of mitochondrial DNA. *Adv. Exp. Med. Biol.* **2012**, *942*, 39–51.
11. Dorstyn, L.; Akey, C.W.; Kumar, S. New insights into apoptosome structure and function. *Cell Death Differ.* **2018**, *25*, 1194–1208. [CrossRef]
12. Kale, J.; Osterlund, E.; Andrews, D. BCL-2 family proteins: Changing partners in the dance towards death. *Cell Death Differ.* **2018**, *25*, 65–80. [CrossRef]
13. Fernández-Silva, P.; Enriquez, J.A.; Montoya, J. Replication and transcription of mammalian mitochondrial DNA. *Exp. Physiol.* **2003**, *88*, 41–56. [CrossRef]
14. Cruz-Zaragoza, L.D.; Dennerlein, S.; Linden, A.; Yousefi, R.; Lavdovskaia, E.; Aich, A.; Falk, R.R.; Gomkale, R.; Schöndorf, T.; Bohnsack, M.T.; et al. An in vitro system to silence mitochondrial gene expression. *Cell* **2021**, *184*, 5824–5837.e15. [CrossRef]
15. Nicholls, T.J.; Minczuk, M. In D-loop: 40 years of mitochondrial 7S DNA. *Exp. Gerontol.* **2014**, *56*, 175–181. [CrossRef]
16. Syndercombe Court, D. Mitochondrial DNA in forensic use. *Emerg. Top Life Sci.* **2021**, *5*, 415–426. [CrossRef]
17. Liu, V.W.; Yang, H.J.; Wang, Y.; Tsang, P.C.K.; Cheung, A.N.; Chiu, P.M.; Ng, T.Y.; Wong, L.C.; Nagley, P.; Ngan, H.Y. High frequency of mitochondrial genome instability in human endometrial carcinomas. *Br. J. Cancer* **2003**, *89*, 697–701. [CrossRef]
18. Genova, M.L.; Bianchi, C.; Lenaz, G. Supercomplex organization of the mitochondrial respiratory chain and the role of the Coenzyme Q pool: Pathophysiological implications. *Biofactors* **2005**, *25*, 5–20. [CrossRef]
19. Kowalczyk, P.; Sulejczak, D.; Kleczkowska, P.; Bukowska-Ośko, I.; Kucia, M.; Popiel, M.; Wietrak, E.; Kramkowski, K.; Wrzosek, K.; Kaczyńska, K. Mitochondrial Oxidative Stress—A Causative Factor and Therapeutic Target in Many Diseases. *Int. J. Mol. Sci.* **2021**, *22*, 13384. [CrossRef]
20. Dabravolski, S.A.; Khotina, V.A.; Sukhorukov, V.N.; Kalmykov, V.A.; Mikhaleva, L.M.; Orekhov, A.N. The Role of Mitochondrial DNA Mutations in Cardiovascular Diseases. *Int. J. Mol. Sci.* **2022**, *23*, 952. [CrossRef]
21. Al-Ghamdi, B.A.; Al-Shamrani, J.M.; El-Shehawi, A.M.; Al-Johani, I.; Al-Otaibi, B.G. Role of mitochondrial DNA in diabetes Mellitus Type I and Type II. *Saudi J. Biol. Sci.* **2022**, *29*, 103434. [CrossRef] [PubMed]
22. Andres, M.P.; Cardena, M.M.S.G.; Fridman, C.; Podgaec, S. Polymorphisms of mitochondrial DNA control region are associated to endometriosis. *J. Assist. Reprod. Genet.* **2018**, *35*, 533–538. [CrossRef] [PubMed]
23. Le Gall, J.Y.; Ardaillou, R. The biology of aging. *Bull. Acad. Natl. Med.* **2009**, *193*, 365. [PubMed]
24. Lujan, S.A.; Longley, M.J.; Humble, M.H.; Lavender, C.A.; Burkholder, A.; Blakely, E.L.; Alston, C.L.; Gorman, G.S.; Turnbull, D.M.; McFarland, R.; et al. Ultrasensitive deletion detection links mitochondrial DNA replication, disease, and aging. *Genome Biol.* **2020**, *21*, 248. [CrossRef] [PubMed]

25. Giorgi, C.; Marchi, S.; Simoes, I.C.M.; Ren, Z.; Morciano, G.; Perrone, M.; Patalas-Krawczyk, P.; Borchard, S.; Jędrak, P.; Pierzynowska, K.; et al. Mitochondria and Reactive Oxygen Species in Aging and Age-Related Diseases. *Int. Rev. Cell Mol. Biol.* **2018**, *340*, 209–344. [CrossRef]
26. Rossmann, M.P.; Dubois, S.M.; Agarwal, S.; Zon, L.I. Mitochondrial function in development and disease. *Dis. Model. Mech.* **2021**, *14*, dmm048912. [CrossRef]
27. Williams, B.; Mancia, G.; Spiering, W.; Agabiti Rosei, E.; Azizi, M.; Burnier, M.; Clement, D.L.; Coca, A.; de Simone, G.; Dominiczak, A.; et al. 2018 ESC/ESH Guidelines for the management of arterial hypertension. *Eur. Heart J.* **2019**, *39*, 3021–3104, Erratum in **2019**, *40*, 475. [CrossRef]
28. Warowicka, A.; Kwasniewska, A.; Gozdzicka-Jozefiak, A. Alterations in mtDNA: A qualitative and quantitative study associated with cervical cancer development. *Gynecol. Oncol.* **2013**, *129*, 193–198. [CrossRef]
29. Available online: http://www.mitomap.org/bin/view.pl/MITOMAP/GenomeLoci (accessed on 9 May 2019).
30. Available online: https://ec.europa.eu/eurostat/statistics-explained/index.php?title=Population_structure_and_ageing#Past_and_future_population_ageing_trends_in_the_EU (accessed on 31 January 2023).
31. McKinney, B.C.; Oh, H.; Sibille, E. Age-by-disease biological interactions: Implications for late-life depression. *Front. Genet.* **2012**, *3*, 237–267. [CrossRef]
32. Pennica, D.; Nedwin, G.E.; Hayflick, J.S.; Seeburg, P.H.; Derynck, R.; Palladino, M.A.; Kohr, W.J.; Aggarwal, B.B.; Goeddel, D.V. Human tumour necrosis factor: Precursor structure, expression and homology to lymphotoxin. *Nature* **1984**, *312*, 724–729. [CrossRef]
33. Troulinaki, K.; Bano, D. Mitochondrial deficiency: A double-edged sword for aging and neurodegeneration. *Front. Genet.* **2012**, *3*, 244. [CrossRef]
34. Elliott, H.R.; Samuels, D.C.; Eden, J.A.; Relton, C.L.; Chinnery, P.F. Pathogenic mitochondrial DNA mutations are common in the general population. *Am. J. Hum. Genet.* **2008**, *83*, 254–260. [CrossRef]
35. Barja, G. Aging in vertebrates, and the effect of caloric restriction: A mitochondrial free radical production-DNA damage mechanism? *Biol. Rev. Camb. Philos. Soc.* **2004**, *79*, 235–251. [CrossRef]
36. Larsen, N.B.; Rasmussen, M.; Rasmussen, L.J. Nuclear and mitochondrial DNA repair: Similar pathways? *Mitochondrion* **2005**, *5*, 89–108. [CrossRef]
37. Michikawa, Y.; Mazzucchelli, F.; Bresolin, N.; Scarlato, G.; Attardi, G. Aging-dependent large accumulation of point mutations in the human mtDNA control region for replication. *Science* **1999**, *286*, 774–779. [CrossRef]
38. Nguyen, D.; Samson, S.L.; Reddy, V.T.; Gonzalez, E.V.; Sekhar, R.V. Impaired mitochondrial fatty acid oxidation and insulin resistance in aging: Novel protective role of glutathione. *Aging Cell.* **2013**, *12*, 415–425. [CrossRef]
39. Yang, C.; Aye, C.C.; Li, X.; Diaz Ramos, A.; Zorzano, A.; Mora, S. Mitochondrial dysfunction in insulin resistance: Differential contributions of chronic insulin and saturated fatty acid exposure in muscle cells. *Biosci. Rep.* **2012**, *32*, 465–478. [CrossRef]
40. Liochev, S.I. Reactive oxygen species and the free radical theory of aging. *Free. Radic. Biol. Med.* **2013**, *60C*, 1–4. [CrossRef]
41. Wei, Y.H.; Lu, C.Y.; Wei, C.Y.; Ma, Y.S.; Lee, H.C. Oxidative stress in human aging and mitochondrial disease-consequences of defective mitochondrial respiration and impaired antioxidant enzyme system. *Chin. J. Physiol.* **2001**, *44*, 1–11.
42. Kokaze, A.; Ishikawa, M.; Matsunaga, N.; Yoshida, M.; Makita, R.; Satoh, M.; Teruya, K.; Sekiguchi, K.; Masuda, Y.; Harada, M.; et al. Longevity-associated mitochondrial DNA 5178 C/A polymorphism is associated with fasting plasma glucose levels and glucose tolerance in Japanese men. *Mitochondrion* **2005**, *5*, 418–425. [CrossRef]
43. Mukae, S.; Aoki, S.; Itoh, S.; Sato, R.; Nishio, K.; Iwata, T.; Katagiri, T. Mitochondrial 5178A/C genotype is associated with acute myocardial infarction. *Circ. J.* **2003**, *67*, 16–20. [CrossRef] [PubMed]
44. Zhang, J.; Asin-Cayuela, J.; Fish, J.; Michikawa, Y.; Bonafe, M.; Olivieri, F.; Passarino, G.; De Benedictis, G.; Franceschi, C.; Attardi, G. Strikingly higher frequency in centenarians and twins of mtDNA mutation causing remodeling of replication origin in leukocytes. *Proc. Natl. Acad. Sci. USA* **2003**, *100*, 1116–1121. [CrossRef] [PubMed]
45. Howell, N.; Elson, J.E.; Howell, C.; Turnbull, D.M. Relative rates of evolution in the coding and control regions of African mtDNAs. *Mol. Biol. Evol.* **2007**, *24*, 2213–2221. [CrossRef]
46. Ingman, M.; Gyllensten, U. mtDB: Human Mitochondrial Genome Database, a resource for population genetics and medical sciences. *Nucleic Acids Res.* **2006**, *34*, D749–D751. [CrossRef] [PubMed]
47. Del Bo, R.; Bordoni, A.; Martinelli Boneschi, F.; Crimi, M.; Sciacco, M.; Bresolin, N.; Scarlato, G.; Comi, G.P. Evidence and age-related distribution of mtDNA D-loop point mutations in skeletal muscle from healthy subjects and mitochondrial patients. *J. Neurol. Sci.* **2002**, *202*, 85–91. [CrossRef] [PubMed]
48. Rydzanicz, M.; Wróbel, M.; Cywińska, K.; Froehlich, D.; Gawecki, W.; Szyfter, W.; Szyfter, K. Screening of the general Polish population for deafness-associated mutations in mitochondrial 12S rRNA and tRNA Ser(UCN) genes. *Genet. Test. Mol. Biomark.* **2009**, *13*, 167–172. [CrossRef]
49. Bray, A.W.; Ballinger, S.W. Mitochondrial DNA mutations and cardiovascular disease. *Curr. Opin. Cardiol.* **2017**, *32*, 267–274. [CrossRef]
50. Litvinova, L.; Zatolokin, P.; Vulf, M.; Mazunin, I.; Skuratovskaia, D. The relationship between the mtDNA copy number in insulin-dependent tissues and markers of endothelial dysfunction and inflammation in obese patients. *BMC Med. Genom.* **2019**, *12* (Suppl. S2), 41. [CrossRef]

51. Ryzhkova, A.I.; Sazonova, M.A.; Sinyov, V.V.; Galitsyna, E.V.; Chicheva, M.M.; Melnichenko, A.A.; Grechko, A.V.; Postnov, A.Y.; Orekhov, A.N.; Shkurat, T.P. Mitochondrial diseases caused by mtDNA mutations: A mini-review. *Ther. Clin. Risk Manag.* **2018**, *14*, 1933–1942. [CrossRef]
52. Jackson, C.B.; Turnbull, D.M.; Minczuk, M.; Gammage, P.A. Therapeutic Manipulation of mtDNA Heteroplasmy: A Shifting Perspective. *Trends Mol. Med.* **2020**, *26*, 698–709. [CrossRef]
53. Pejovic, T.; Ladner, D.; Intengan, M.; Zheng, K.; Fairchild, T.; Dillon, D.; Easley, S.; Dillon, D.; Marchetti, D.; Schwartz, P. Somatic D-loop mitochondrialDNA mutations are frequent in uterine serous carcinoma. *Eur. J. Cancer* **2004**, *40*, 2519–2524. [CrossRef]
54. Dikalov, S.I.; Dikalova, A.E. Contribution of mitochondrial oxidative stress to hypertension. *Curr. Opin. Nephrol. Hypertens.* **2016**, *25*, 73–80. [CrossRef]
55. Rubanyi, G.M.; Vanhoutte, P.M. Superoxide anions and hyperoxia inactivate endothelium-derived relaxing factor. *Am. J. Physiol.* **1986**, *250*, 822–827. [CrossRef]
56. Pryor, W.A.; Squadrito, G.L. The chemistry of peroxynitrite: A product from the reaction of nitric oxide with superoxide. *Am. J. Physiol.* **1995**, *268*, 699–722. [CrossRef]
57. Liu, Y.; Li, R.; Li, Z.; Wang, X.J.; Yang, L.; Wang, S.; Guan, M.X. Mitochondrial transfer RNAMet 4435A>G mutation is associated with maternally inherited hypertension in a Chinese pedigree. *Hypertension* **2009**, *53*, 1083–1090. [CrossRef]
58. Wang, S.; Li, R.; Fettermann, A.; Li, Z.; Qian, Y.; Liu, Y.; Wang, X.; Zhou, A.; Mo, J.Q.; Yang, L.; et al. Maternally inherited essential hypertension is associated with the novel 4263A>G mutation in the mitochondrial tRNAIle gene in a large Han Chinese family. *Circ. Res.* **2011**, *108*, 862–870. [CrossRef]
59. Li, R.; Liu, Y.; Li, Z.; Yang, L.; Wang, S.; Guan, M.X. Failures in mitochondrial tRNAMet and tRNAGln metabolism caused by the novel 4401A>G mutation are involved in essential hypertension in a Han Chinese Family. *Hypertension* **2009**, *54*, 329–337. [CrossRef]
60. Lu, C.Q.; Zhang, J.Y.; Xu, A.G.; Zhang, J.J.; Li, D.D.; Fu, X.; Guo, J.; Xu, Q.F. Mitochondrial tRNAMet mutation is associated with clinical and biochemical characteristics in primary hypertension. *Mol. Med. Rep.* **2013**, *7*, 1924–1928. [CrossRef]
61. Liu, Y.; Li, Z.; Yang, L.; Wang, S.; Guan, M.X. The mitochondrial ND1 T3308C mutation in a Chinese family with the secondary hypertension. *Biochem. Biophys. Res. Commun.* **2008**, *368*, 18–22. [CrossRef]
62. Liu, L.L.; Tan, D.J.; Wang, S.W.; Wong, L.J. Evaluation of inheritable character in essential hypertension through reconstruction of neighbor-joining tree. *Yi Chuan* **2004**, *26*, 441–445.
63. Shoji, M.; Tsutaya, S.; Kasai, T.; Yasujima, M. Implication of single nucleotide polymorphisms in association study: Mitochondrial variations as another genetic markers for hypertension. *Rinsho Byori.* **2002**, *50*, 497–501. [PubMed]

biomedicines

Article

The Involvement of Endogenous Enkephalins in Glucose Homeostasis †

Vanessa Escolero [1,2], Laica Tolentino [1], Abdul Bari Muhammad [1,3], Abdul Hamid [4] and Kabirullah Lutfy [4,*]

1 Graduate College of Biomedical Sciences, Western University of Health Sciences, Pomona, CA 91766, USA
2 Burrell College of Osteopathic Medicine, 3501 Arrowhead Drive, Las Cruces, NM 88001, USA
3 Cardiovascular and Metabolism (CVM), Janssen Research and Development, 100 Binney Street, 5th Floor, Cambridge, MA 02141, USA
4 Department of Pharmaceutical Sciences, College of Pharmacy, Western University of Health Sciences, Pomona, CA 91766, USA
* Correspondence: klutfy@westernu.edu
† This study was a part of VE's thesis project; A.B.M. and K.L. served as co-mentors.

Abstract: Obesity has nearly tripled since 1975 and is predicted to continue to escalate. The surge in obesity is expected to increase the risk of diabetes type 2, hypertension, coronary artery disease, and stroke. Therefore, it is essential to better understand the mechanisms that regulate energy and glucose homeostasis. The opioid system is implicated in regulating both aspects (hedonic and homeostatic) of food intake. Specifically, in the present study, we investigated the role of endogenous enkephalins in changes in food intake and glucose homeostasis. We used preproenkephalin (ppENK) knockout mice and their wildtype littermates/controls to assess changes in body weight, food intake, and plasma glucose levels when mice were fed a high-fat diet for 16 weeks. Body weight and food intake were measured every week (n = 21–23 mice per genotype), and at the end of the 16-week exposure period, mice were tested using the oral glucose tolerance test (OGTT, n = 9 mice per genotype) and insulin tolerance test (n = 5 mice per genotype). Our results revealed no difference in body weight or food intake between mice of the two genotypes. However, HFD-exposed enkephalin-deficient mice demonstrated impaired OGTT associated with reduced insulin sensitivity compared to their wildtype controls. The impaired insulin sensitivity is possibly due to the development of peripheral insulin resistance. Our results reveal a potential role of enkephalins in the regulation of glucose homeostasis and in the pathophysiology of diabetes type 2.

Keywords: enkephalins; high-fat diet (HFD); obesity/diabetes type 2; oral glucose tolerance test (GTT); insulin tolerance test (ITT)

1. Introduction

Worldwide obesity has nearly tripled since 1975, and current trends are expected to continue to rise [1]. As per World Health Organization (WHO) 2022 statistics, more than 1 billion people are obese worldwide [2]. In addition, a recent report from the Center for Disease Control (CDC) estimated that the prevalence of obesity from 2017 to 2020 in the United States was 41.9% among adults and 19.7% among children and adolescents [3]. The increased rates of obesity are driven primarily by the overconsumption of energy-dense foods and an increase in sedentary lifestyles, resulting in a shift in energy balance that leads to excessive fat accumulation. Furthermore, this increases the risks for chronic comorbidities such as diabetes type 2, coronary artery disease, hypertension, stroke, and certain cancers [4]. Given the continued rise in obesity and diabetes type 2 over the past decades, understanding the mechanisms that regulate energy homeostasis and glucose metabolism would be beneficial in developing novel therapeutics to prevent or at least reduce the devastating public health and socioeconomic consequences of obesity and diabetes type 2.

The endogenous opioid system, consisting of opioid peptides (beta-endorphin, dynorphin, and enkephalins) and their corresponding G-protein-coupled receptors, namely, delta (DOP), kappa (KOP), and mu (MOP) opioid receptors [5,6], is heavily implicated in feeding behavior. These opioid peptides and their receptors are highly expressed in brain regions involved in the rewarding and hedonic aspects of feeding, such as the mesolimbic dopaminergic system. In addition, these opioid peptides are localized within the hypothalamus and, thus, are likely involved in modulating homeostatic signals received from the peripheral tissues [7]. Pharmacological studies have shown that opioid receptor agonists stimulate food intake [8,9], while opioid receptor antagonists suppress food intake [8,10,11]. However, the role of each opioid peptide in feeding behavior and, notably, glucose homeostasis is not fully understood.

Previous studies have shown that the administration of enkephalin and enkephalin analogs increases the intake of palatable food [12,13]. Moreover, an increase in enkephalin mRNA was observed in the brain of rats consuming a high-fat diet, reinforcing a positive relationship between a high-fat diet and enkephalin [13]. In addition, a 2015 study showed that mice lacking the ability to produce enkephalin gained less weight when compared to their wildtype controls despite equal amounts of food intake [14].

Enkephalins are found in several peripheral organs, including the pancreas, liver, adipose, skeletal muscle, lungs, heart, as well as in the central and peripheral nervous systems, suggesting the involvement of enkephalins in various biological processes such as feeding behavior [15]. Indeed, enkephalins have been shown to play a functional role in glucose metabolism. For example, one of the first studies conducted in the 1980s demonstrated the presence of opioid receptors in the islets and a low dose of enkephalin-stimulated insulin secretion in vitro [16]. In contrast, in vitro high concentrations of enkephalin inhibited insulin release [16,17], raising the possibility that enkephalins may regulate insulin secretion and glucose homeostasis. Interestingly, delta-opioid-receptor-deficient mice fed a chow diet demonstrated improved glucose tolerance compared to wildtype; however, when challenged with a high-fat diet, the difference between genotypes disappeared [18]. Most recently, enkephalins have been implicated in the beiging process of white adipocytes through the activation of group 2 innate lymphoid cells [19]. However, the role of enkephalins is partially characterized in feeding and glucose homeostasis. Therefore, our study aims to further understand the role of the opioid peptides, enkephalins, in the regulation of body weight and glucose homeostasis.

2. Materials and Methods

2.1. Animals

We utilized enkephalin knockout mice that were previously generated by Konig and colleagues [20]. Mice lacking the preproenkephalin (ppENK) gene and their wildtype controls were fully backcrossed on a C57BL/6 mouse strain and bred in-house. Pups were weaned on day 21 and genotyped according to our earlier reports [21,22]. In total, there were 21 wildtype and 19 knockout male mice used, but 2 wildtype and 2 knockout mice were sacrificed early in the experiment due to severe dermatitis and excluded from the data analysis. Mice were housed in recyclable plastic cages with bedding and ad libitum access to food and water under a 12 h light/12 h dark cycle in a temperature- and humidity-controlled room. Animal cages were changed to new cages every two weeks. All animal experiments were performed in accordance with the NIH guideline for the care and use of animals in research and approved by the Western University of Health Sciences Institutional Animal Care and Use Committee (Pomona, CA, USA), protocol number R20IACUC024.

2.2. Diet

Mice were maintained on a regular laboratory chow diet (Envigo Teklad Global Diets, 2018, 18% protein rodent diet; 24% kcal protein, 18% kcal fat, and 58% kcal carbohydrates; 3.1 kcal/g) for one week. Then, for the remainder of the study, mice were placed on a high-fat diet obtained from Research Diets, Inc (60% kcal fat, 20% kcal carbohydrates, and 20% kcal protein with blue dye: 5.21 kcal/g formulation D12492).

2.3. The Role of Enkephalins in Body Weight and Food Intake

To determine the involvement of endogenous enkephalins in body weight and food intake, we used mice lacking enkephalins and their wildtype littermates/controls that we described previously [21,22]. The experiment was conducted over the course of 17 weeks. Each animal had their body weight and food intake measured in grams (g), once weekly. Initially, animals were isolated and housed one per cage and given a regular diet for the first week to habituate to a single mouse per cage condition. This was performed to enable us to measure the food intake of each mouse accurately and also to avoid fighting in the cage, as this can be stressful and affect food intake and importantly blood glucose. At week 2, they were switched to the high-fat diet (HFD) and remained on the HFD through week 17. The experiment was repeated four times with 4–6 mice per cohort (n = 21–23 mice per genotype).

2.4. The Role of Enkephalins in Glucose Homeostasis

To determine the role of enkephalin in glucose homeostasis, an oral glucose tolerance test (OGTT) was conducted at week 17 in 2 different sets (n = 3–5 mice per cohort) of mice (n = 8 mice per genotype). The protocol was according to our earlier report [23]. Mice were fasted overnight starting at 10 p.m., for a total of 11 h with ad libitum access to water during this period. The next morning (9 AM), while the animals were still kept fasted, a small piece of the tail was snipped, and the baseline blood glucose level was measured for each mouse, using a glucometer (Embrace Omnis Blood Glucose Monitoring System/Omnis Health Embrace Blood Glucose Test Strip). Mice were then weighed and administered a 2 g/kg of glucose solution via oral gavage. Blood glucose levels were then measured at 30, 60, 90, 120 min after the glucose challenge. At the end of the experiment, mice were restored with ad libitum access to water and food.

2.5. The Role of Enkephalins in Insulin Sensitivity

To determine the role of enkephalins in insulin sensitivity and provide complementary results to the glucose tolerance test, a separate set of mice underwent an intraperitoneal insulin tolerance test (ITT) at week 17. The ITT protocol was according to our earlier report, except we fasted the mice for 6 h to avoid hypoglycemia [23]. Briefly, mice were kept fasted for a total of 6 h with access to ad libitum water. Mice were weighed and then given 0.75 U/kg insulin intraperitoneally (Humulin R 100 U/mL, Eli Lilly and Company). Tail vein blood was used to measure blood glucose levels using a glucometer, as described above. Blood glucose levels were measured before (time 0) and at 15, 30, 45, 60, 90 min after insulin injection. At the end of the experiment, mice were restored with ad libitum access to water and food.

2.6. The Role of Enkephalin in Plasma Insulin Levels

Considering changes in plasma insulin level can alter blood glucose levels, we also assessed if the lack of enkephalins would alter plasma insulin levels. Briefly, mice (n = 8–10 mice per genotype) were euthanatized through decapitation. Whole trunk blood was collected in ethylenediaminetetraacetic acid (EDTA)-containing tubes and centrifuged at 14,000 rpm for 10 min at 4 °C. Plasma samples were collected and stored in a −80 °C freezer until analysis. Mouse insulin levels were measured with a commercially available ELISA kit (Rat/Mouse Insulin ELISA Kit, Cat. # EZRMI-13K). The protocol supplied by the kit manufacturer was followed. Briefly, a 96-well plate pre-coated with monoclonal mouse anti-rat insulin antibodies was loaded with six rat insulin standards, two quality controls, background, and samples. Each sample was diluted 2-fold with the assay buffer according to the manufacturer's instructions and run in duplicates. The absorbance was read at a wavelength of 450 nm with a plate reader. Based on the standard curves run in duplicate on each plate, plasma insulin concentration was determined with linear regression using GraphPad Prism 9.1.2 software (San Diego, CA, USA).

2.7. The Role of Enkephalin in Plasma Leptin Levels

Given that changes in leptin levels can affect plasma glucose levels, we also examined if the lack of enkephalins would alter plasma leptin levels. Mice (n = 9–11 per genotype) were euthanized, and trunk blood was corrected and prepared, as described above. Mouse leptin levels were measured with a commercially available ELISA kit (Mouse Leptin ELISA Kit, Cat. # EZML-82K). The protocol supplied by the kit manufacturer was followed. Briefly, a 96-well plate pre-coated with pre-tittered antiserum was loaded with six rat insulin standards, two quality controls, background, and samples. Each sample was analyzed in duplicates and diluted 2-fold with assay buffer according to the manufacturer's instructions. The absorbance was read at a wavelength of 450 nm with a plate reader. Based on the standard curves run in duplicate on each plate, plasma leptin concentration was determined with linear regression using GraphPad Prism 9.1.2 software (San Diego, CA, USA).

2.8. Statistical Analysis

Data were expressed as mean ± SEM. Time-course data were analyzed using two-way repeated measures analysis of variance (ANOVA) followed by Fisher's LSD post hoc multiple comparisons. The area under the curve (AUC) for the OGTT and ITT time-course data was calculated using the trapezoidal rule. Plasma insulin and leptin levels were measured using linear regression analysis. A *p*-value < 0.05 was considered significant. Statistical analysis and graphing were completed in GraphPad Prism version 9 (San Diego, CA, USA).

3. Results

3.1. Body Wight Measurement in Wildtype and Knockout Mice

We first determined if endogenous enkephalins regulate body weight. Figure 1 shows the raw body weight of male wildtype (ppENK+/+) and knockout (ppENK-/-) animals for the duration of the experiment. The knockout mice displayed a similar pattern in body weight gain as the wildtype mice. A mixed-effects analysis revealed a significant effect for time ($p < 0.0001$) but no effect for genotype ($p = 0.9673$) or genotype x time ($p = 0.9946$). The percentage change in body weight was also not different between the wildtype and knockout animals (Figure 1b). A mixed-effects analysis revealed a significant effect for time ($p < 0.0001$) but not for genotype ($p = 0.0136$) or genotype x time ($p = 0.1714$). This result reveals that endogenous enkephalins may not play a significant role in HFD-induced weight gain.

3.2. Food Intake Measurement in Wildtype and Knockout Mice

To assess if endogenous enkephalins alter food intake, we used mice lacking enkephalins and their wildtype littermates. Figure 2 shows the daily food intake in grams (g) between wildtype and knockout animals fed the regular and HFD. Week 1 demonstrates the initial measurement of the regular diet (g) followed by the HFD on week 2, as marked on the graph. As can be observed, there was a drop in daily food intake from week 1 to week 2, likely due to the HFD containing higher total calories than the regular diet, leading to reduced consumption. However, there were no significant differences in food intake between wildtype and knockout mice. A mixed-effects analysis revealed a significant effect for time ($p < 0.0001$) but no effect for genotype ($p = 1.023$) or genotype x time ($p = 0.6778$). This result suggests that endogenous enkephalins may not regulate regular diet or HFD consumption.

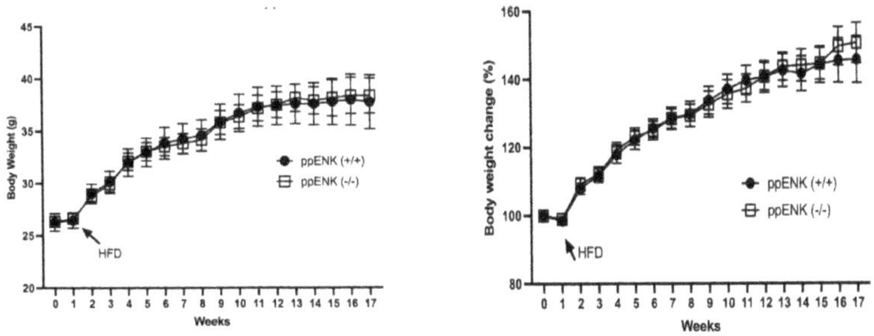

(a) (b)

Figure 1. Body weight changes in mice lacking enkephalins (ppENK-/-) and their wildtype (ppENK+/+) littermates on HFD for 16 weeks. Data represent mean (±S.E.M.) of raw body weight (**a**) and percent of change in the original weight of mice of each genotype (**b**). The experiment was repeated four times with 5–7 mice per cohort (n = 21–23 mice per genotype). No significant difference was observed in either parameter between mice of the two genotypes ($p > 0.05$).

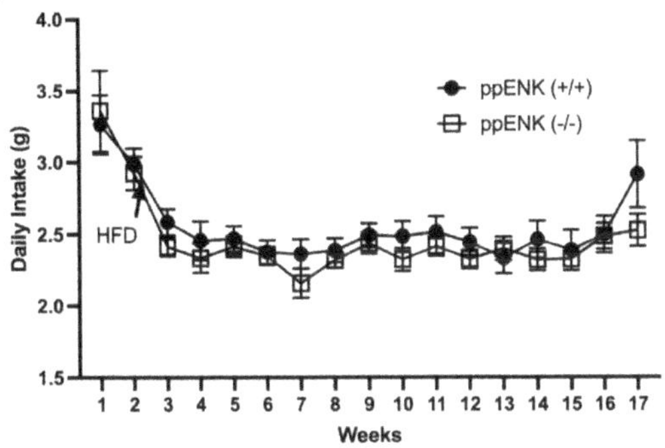

Figure 2. Changes in food intake in mice lacking enkephalins (ppENK-/-) and their wildtype (ppENK+/+) littermates when placed on HFD for 16 weeks. Data represent mean (±S.E.M.) of food intake (g) measured once a week for a total of 16 weeks in mice of the two genotypes. The experiment was repeated four times with 5–7 mice per cohort (n = 21–23 mice per genotype). No significant difference was observed in food intake between mice of the two genotypes ($p > 0.05$).

3.3. Oral Glucose Tolerance Test

To examine the role of enkephalin in glucose homeostasis, an oral glucose tolerance test (OGTT) was conducted in mice lacking enkephalins and their wildtype littermates. The study was repeated twice with n = 4–5 per cohort (n = 9 mice per genotype). Briefly, the mice were fasted overnight, and fasted blood glucose levels were measured before administering a glucose solution via oral gavage. Subsequently, a 2 g/kg oral glucose gavage was administered, and blood glucose levels (mg/dL) were measured between wildtype and knockout mice at specific time points for a total of 90 min, as shown in Figure 3. We observed glucose intolerance in ppENK knockout mice throughout all time points after oral gavage compared to wildtype mice. A two-way ANOVA analysis revealed a significant effect for time ($F(3, 48) = 57.42$, $p < 0.0001$), genotype ($F(1, 16) = 7.106$, $p = 0.0169$), but no interaction between time x genotype ($F(3, 48) = 1.013$, $p = 0.3953$). Fisher's LSD post hoc test revealed a significant increase at 30 and 60 min in mice lacking enkephalin compared to the wildtype. An unpaired student's *t*-test of the AUC also showed a significant ($p < 0.02$) increase in blood glucose levels in mice lacking enkephalins compared to their wildtype controls (t = 2.84, df = 16; Figure 3b). This rise could be due to changes in basal fasting glucose between wildtype and knockout mice. While repeated measures ANOVA did not reveal any significant difference in basal fasting glucose between mice of the two genotypes, this was a significant difference when basal levels were analyzed by unpaired student's t-test ($t = 2.41$; df = 16; $p < 0.02$). However, this difference was not observed when animals were fasted for 6 h for the ITT (see below). These results suggest that glucose handling in the absence of enkephalins is reduced. However, basal fasting glucose is only affected when the duration of fasting is 12 h.

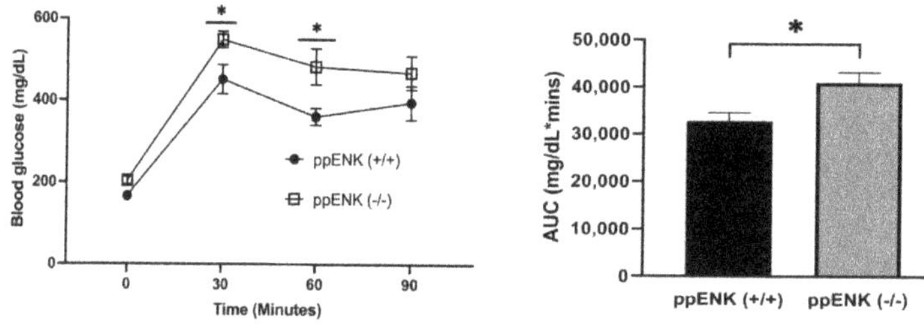

(a) (b)

Figure 3. Oral glucose tolerance test (OGTT) performed after overnight fasting in mice lacking enkephalins (ppENK-/-) and their wildtype (ppENK+/+) littermates placed on HFD for 16 weeks. Data represent mean (±S.E.M.) of blood glucose levels (mg/dl) measured before and 30, 60, and 90 min after an oral glucose (2 g/kg, p.o.) challenge (**a**) and AUC (**b**). The experiment was repeated two times with 4–5 mice per cohort (n = 9 mice per genotype). * $p < 0.05$ a significant difference between mice of the two genotypes by Fisher's LSD test (**a**) or unpaired student's t-test (**b**).

3.4. Insulin Tolerance Test

We conducted an insulin tolerance test to determine whether the impaired glucose tolerance in the knockout than wildtype mice was due to reduced sensitivity to insulin. In total there were seven ppENK wildtype (ppENK+/+) and five knockout (ppENK-/-) male mice; however, two wildtype mice were excluded from the analysis, as these mice were non-responsive to the insulin challenge. The blood glucose levels of these mice remained elevated throughout the experiment compared to the rest. Briefly, mice were kept fasted for 6 h, and fasting blood glucose levels were measured before the intraperitoneal insulin injection. Following a 0.75 U/Kg insulin injection was administered intraperitoneally, blood glucose levels (mg/dL) were measured and compared between wildtype and knockout for 90 min, as shown in Figure 4. We observed knockout mice were glucose-intolerant at all time points following the insulin injection. These findings were consistent with the OGTT results, demonstrating that ppENK-deficient mice have reduced glucose tolerance and are insulin resistant. A two-way ANOVA analysis demonstrated a significant effect of time ($F(5, 40) = 11.70$, $p < 0.0001$), genotype ($F(1, 8) = 11.08$, $p = 0.0104$), but no interaction between time x genotype ($F(5, 40) = 1.090$, $p = 0.3806$). The Fisher's LSD test revealed that there was a significant increase in blood glucose at 45 and 90 min in knockout mice compared to their wildtype controls. Analyses of the AUC also revealed a significant ($p < 0.01$) increase in blood glucose in mice lacking enkephalins than their wildtype littermates ($t = 3.60$; df = 8; Figure 4b). These results suggest that insulin sensitivity is impaired in mice lacking enkephalins following exposure to HFD for 16 weeks.

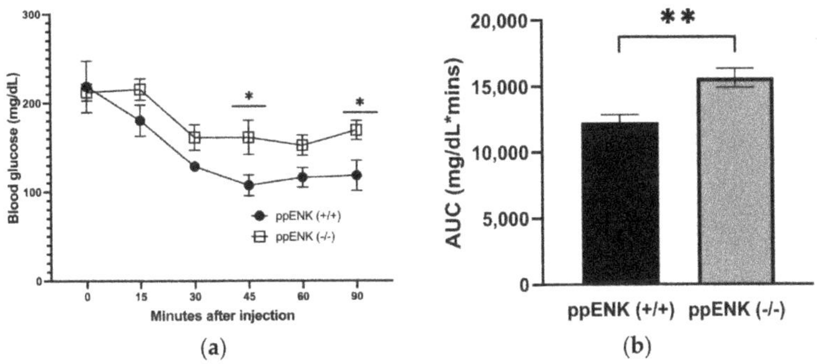

Figure 4. Insulin tolerance test (ITT) performed after six hours of fasting in mice lacking enkephalins (ppENK-/-) and their wildtype (ppENK+/+) littermates exposed to HFD for 16 weeks. Data represent mean (±S.E.M.) of blood glucose levels (mg/dL) measured before and 30, 60, and 90 min after an insulin (0.75 g/kg, i.p.) challenge (**a**) and calculated AUC (**b**) in wildtype and knockout mice (n = 5 mice per genotype). A significant difference between mice of the two genotypes by the Fisher's LSD test (* $p < 0.05$, panel (**a**)) or unpaired student's t-test (** $p < 0.01$, panel (**b**)).

3.5. Insulin and Leptin Measurement in Wildtype and Knockout Mice

We then investigated if enkephalins could also regulate the level of insulin or leptin, which could explain the changes observed in the OGTT and ITT. We measured the plasma insulin and leptin levels through enzyme-linked immunosorbent assay (ELISA) using a commercially available ELISA kit in wildtype and knockout mice. As shown in Figure 5a, the plasma insulin levels were comparable in wildtype and knockout mice. An unpaired student's t-test was utilized for statistical analysis, which revealed no significance (t(df = 16) = 0.3155, $p = 0.7565$). In addition, plasma leptin levels were also measured utilizing a commercially available ELISA kit. As shown in Figure 5b, there were no significant differences in plasma leptin between wildtype and knockout mice. For statistical analysis, an unpaired student's t-test was used, which demonstrated no significance (t(df = 16) = 0.2194, $p = 0.8288$). This result shows that enkephalins may not regulate plasma insulin or leptin levels in mice exposed to HFD for 16 weeks.

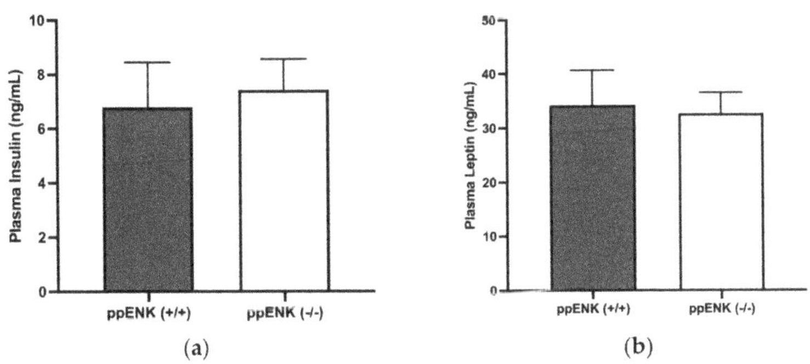

Figure 5. Plasma levels of insulin (**a**) and leptin (**b**) in mice lacking enkephalins (ppENK-/-) and their wildtype (ppENK+/+) littermates on HFD for 16 weeks. Data represent mean (±S.E.M.) of plasma levels of insulin ((**a**), 8–10 mice per genotype) and leptin ((**b**), n = 9–11 mice per genotype) in ng/mL. No significant difference was observed in either parameter between mice of the two genotypes ($p > 0.05$).

4. Discussion

The regulation of nutrient intake and metabolism is tightly regulated by the interplay of numerous systems [24,25]. In this study, we focused on the opioid system, specifically the role of enkephalins in food intake and glucose homeostasis. As stated earlier, only a handful of studies have examined the role of enkephalins in energy and glucose homeostasis. The findings in this study are consistent with the literature, demonstrating that opioids play a role in glucose and energy homeostasis; specifically, our study suggests that enkephalins are likely involved in glucose homeostasis.

Our results suggest that the deletion of enkephalins does not affect food intake or body weight, as there was no statistically significant difference in raw body weight or the percentage of body weight changes between mice lacking enkephalins and their wildtype controls. Our results contrast that of Mendez et al. (2015), which was one of the first studies that demonstrated mice lacking enkephalins were resistant to diet-induced obesity compared to wildtype controls, although there was no difference in food consumption between mice of the two genotypes [14]. Enkephalins are implicated in the beiging of white adipocytes through the activation of uncoupling protein-1 (UCP-1) [19]. However, the different diets and the duration of exposure may explain the discrepancy between our results and that of Mendez and colleagues who utilized a "cafeteria diet" composed of snacks, such as cheese puffs, pretzels, cereal, marshmallows, pepperoni, etc. [14]. Age differences should also be investigated as the starting age of animals for our study ranged from 10 to 26 weeks compared to 21 weeks in the former study [14].

Previous studies have shown differences in plasma glucose levels in mice lacking kappa (KOP), mu (MOP), and delta (DOP) compared to their respective wildtype controls [18,26,27]. The current literature demonstrates that MOP knockout mice have enhanced glucose tolerance when fed a high-fat diet, and similar results have been observed in mice lacking DOP or KOP [26–28]. However, the role of each opioid peptide in regulating glucose homeostasis is unclear. Thus, we used mice lacking enkephalins and their wildtype littermates/age-matched controls to assess whether basal or oral glucose tolerance tests would be altered in the absence of enkephalins. We also assessed insulin tolerance test in mice lacking enkephalins and their wildtype littermates/controls to assess if the change in plasma glucose observed in the OGGT is a result of changes in insulin sensitivity. Our data show elevated basal blood glucose levels in mice of both genotypes, which is expected based on the literature and consistent with insulin resistance in mice fed a high-fat diet [29,30]. However, enkephalin knockout mice had higher blood glucose in the OGTT and impaired insulin sensitivity in the ITT compared to their wildtype littermates/controls. These findings suggest that enkephalins may offer protection from the negative effects of a dense, high-fat diet on glucose homeostasis and insulin sensitivity in mice. While the 12 h fasting led to a significant difference in basal glucose levels between wildtype and knockout mice, the 6 h fasting was without any effect on basal glucose level (ITT data). It appears that longer fasting may be necessary to yield a difference in basal fasting glucose levels between wildtype and knockout mice, suggesting that enkephalins may regulate basal glucose levels in mice exposed to HFD for 16 weeks and exposed to 12 h of fasting. On the contrary, enkephalin knockout mice fed a chow diet did not show an impaired glucose tolerance test (Figure S1, Supplemental Data), which is consistent with data obtained in DOP knockout mice fed a regular diet, as they did not show an impaired glucose tolerance test compared to their high-fat-diet-fed wildtype counterparts [18].

In addition, our enkephalin knockout mice demonstrated impaired insulin sensitivity during the insulin tolerance test, indicating elevated glucose levels are possibly due to the development of peripheral insulin resistance. It needs to be noted that the rise in glucose could also be due to reduced insulin release from the pancreas. However, the measured plasma insulin levels showed no significant difference between mice of the two genotypes. Additionally, no change in plasma leptin was found between wildtype and knockout mice, but further studies are needed to comprehensively assess the role of enkephalins in plasma insulin and leptin regulation. At the time of blood collection, our mice were not fasted, which likely contributed to the measured results. Additionally, the mice were not challenged with glucose, which allowed us to measure glucose-stimulated insulin secretion. Therefore, repeating this experiment using glucose-stimulated insulin secretion (GSIS) will provide useful information concerning the role of enkephalins in regulating insulin secretion. Regardless, the OGTT and ITT do indicate that these mice are insulin-resistant.

Enkephalins are widely distributed throughout the brain and various organs. Therefore, it is possible that enkephalins influence mechanisms involved in lipid or glucose metabolism within these tissues [7,18]. Specifically, increased gluconeogenesis in the liver contributes to hyperglycemia in diabetes [31]. Under normal conditions, gluconeogenesis is suppressed in the liver when there is elevated blood glucose. However, the dysregulation of key regulatory enzymes, such as glucose-6 phosphatase or phosphoenolpyruvate carboxylase, may contribute to uncontrolled gluconeogenesis in the presence of hyperglycemia or decreased insulin levels; although in our study, we did not observe any difference in insulin levels between the two genotypes, we measured it a few days after the OGTT and ITT. As stated above, there are several studies utilizing both MOP and DOP knockout mice that show elevated liver enzymes, specifically those involved in fatty acid oxidation. The measured difference in these enzymes between knockout and wildtype mice likely influences the phenotype of these mice when fed an HFD [18,27]. Therefore, future studies need to be designed to measure the level and activity of enzymes, such as acetyl-CoA carboxylase (ACC-α) and peroxisome proliferator-activated receptor (PPAR-α). It is also necessary to further investigate the role of adipose tissue, as Brestoff et al. (2015) demonstrated that beiging through UCP-1 can be modulated by enkephalins [19]. Thus, future studies are also needed to determine the alteration in brown and white adipose tissues in the presence and absence of enkephalin to comprehensively understand the role of enkephalin in the regulation of glucose homeostasis.

5. Conclusions

The opioid system is relatively well known for regulating food consumption and energy homeostasis. In addition to the well-studied opioid receptors, enkephalins may also contribute to energy homeostasis. Our study adds to the current literature by demonstrating that glucose homeostasis is impaired in the absence of enkephalins, and this may be due to reduced insulin sensitivity. However, a great deal of work is needed to better understand the role of enkephalins in this process. We also need to determine the interaction of enkephalins with the neuropeptide systems controlling feeding behavior and glucose homeostasis. Investigating both the central and peripheral effects of enkephalin may reveal how enkephalins alter glucose homeostasis. Considering that we used mice lacking enkephalins throughout the body and throughout their life cycle, additional studies, using pharmacological and molecular biological tools, are needed to temporarily silence the enkephalin gene to have a better understanding of the role of this system in glucose homeostasis.

Supplementary Materials: The following supporting information can be downloaded at: https://www.mdpi.com/article/10.3390/biomedicines11030671/s1, Figure S1: Plasma glucose level was unaltered in the absence of enkephalins in mice fed a regular chow diet.

Author Contributions: Conceptualization, A.B.M. and K.L.; methodology, V.E., A.H. and K.L.; software, V.E. and L.T.; validation, V.E. and K.L.; formal analysis, V.E., L.T. and K.L.; investigation, V.E., A.H. and K.L.; resources, K.L.; data curation, V.E.; writing—original draft preparation, V.E.; writing—review and editing, V.E., L.T., A.B.M. and K.L.; supervision, A.B.M. and K.L.; project administration, K.L. All authors have read and agreed to the published version of the manuscript.

Funding: This research received no external funding.

Institutional Review Board Statement: The study was conducted in accordance with the NIH guideline for the proper use of animals in research and approved by the Institutional Animal Care and Use Committee (R20/IACUC/024).

Informed Consent Statement: Not applicable.

Data Availability Statement: Data will be made available upon reasonable request.

Acknowledgments: The authors wish to thank the Department of Pharmaceutical Sciences, College of Pharmacy, and Graduate College of Biomedical Sciences (GCBS) at Western University of Health Sciences for their support. This study was part of VE's thesis project, on which ABM and KL served as co-mentors, and was submitted in partial fulfillment of the requirements for the degree of Master of Sciences in Biomedical Sciences at GCBS.

Conflicts of Interest: The authors declare no conflict of interest.

References

1. WHO. Obesity and Overweight. Available online: https://www.who.int/news-room/fact-sheets/detail/obesity-and-overweight (accessed on 16 June 2022).
2. Volpi, F. World Obesity Day 2022—Accelerating Action to Stop Obesity. Available online: https://www.who.int/news/item/04-03-2022-world-obesity-day-2022-accelerating-action-to-stop-obesity#:~:text=WHO%20estimates%20that%20by%202025,predictable%20and%20preventable%20health%20crisis (accessed on 25 January 2023).
3. Stierman, B.; Afful, J.; Carroll, M.D.; Chen, T.C.; Davy, O.; Fink, S.; Fryar, C.D.; Gu, Q.; Hales, C.M.; Hughes, J.P.; et al. National Health and Nutrition Examination Survey 2017–March 2020 Prepandemic Data Files Development of Files and Prevalence Estimates for Selected Health Outcomes. *Natl. Health Stat. Rep.* **2021**, *NHSR No. 158*. [CrossRef]
4. Bomberg, E.; Birch, L.; Endenburg, N.; German, A.J.; Neilson, J.; Seligman, H.; Takashima, G.; Day, M.J. The Financial Costs, Behaviour and Psychology of Obesity: A One Health Analysis. *J. Comp. Pathol.* **2017**, *156*, 310–325. [CrossRef]
5. Bodnar, R.J. Endogenous opioid modulation of food intake and body weight: Implications for opioid influences upon motivation and addiction. *Peptides* **2019**, *116*, 42–62. [CrossRef]
6. Pasternak, G.W.; Pan, Y.X. Mu opioids and their receptors: Evolution of a concept. *Pharm. Rev.* **2013**, *65*, 1257–1317. [CrossRef]
7. Nogueiras, R.; Romero-Pico, A.; Vazquez, M.J.; Novelle, M.G.; Lopez, M.; Dieguez, C. The opioid system and food intake: Homeostatic and hedonic mechanisms. *Obes. Facts* **2012**, *5*, 196–207. [CrossRef]
8. Giraudo, S.Q.; Billington, C.J.; Levine, A.S. Effects of the opioid antagonist naltrexone on feeding induced by DAMGO in the central nucleus of the amygdala and in the paraventricular nucleus in the rat. *Brain Res.* **1998**, *782*, 18–23. [CrossRef]
9. Spanagel, R.; Herz, A.; Shippenberg, T.S. Opposing tonically active endogenous opioid systems modulate the mesolimbic dopaminergic pathway. *Proc. Natl. Acad. Sci. USA* **1992**, *89*, 2046–2050. [CrossRef]
10. Levine, A.S.; Weldon, D.T.; Grace, M.; Cleary, J.P.; Billington, C.J. Naloxone blocks that portion of feeding driven by sweet taste in food-restricted rats. *Am. J. Physiol.* **1995**, *268*, R248–R252. [CrossRef]
11. Kanarek, R.B.; Mathes, W.F.; Heisler, L.K.; Lima, R.P.; Monfared, L.S. Prior exposure to palatable solutions enhances the effects of naltrexone on food intake in rats. *Pharm. Biochem. Behav.* **1997**, *57*, 377–381. [CrossRef]
12. Naleid, A.M.; Grace, M.K.; Chimukangara, M.; Billington, C.J.; Levine, A.S. Paraventricular opioids alter intake of high-fat but not high-sucrose diet depending on diet preference in a binge model of feeding. *Am. J. Physiol. Regul. Integr. Comp. Physiol.* **2007**, *293*, R99–R105. [CrossRef]
13. Chang, G.Q.; Karatayev, O.; Barson, J.R.; Chang, S.Y.; Leibowitz, S.F. Increased enkephalin in brain of rats prone to overconsuming a fat-rich diet. *Physiol. Behav.* **2010**, *101*, 360–369. [CrossRef]
14. Mendez, I.A.; Ostlund, S.B.; Maidment, N.T.; Murphy, N.P. Involvement of Endogenous Enkephalins and beta-Endorphin in Feeding and Diet-Induced Obesity. *Neuropsychopharmacology* **2015**, *40*, 2103–2112. [CrossRef]
15. Denning, G.M.; Ackermann, L.W.; Barna, T.J.; Armstrong, J.G.; Stoll, L.L.; Weintraub, N.L.; Dickson, E.W. Proenkephalin expression and enkephalin release are widely observed in non-neuronal tissues. *Peptides* **2008**, *29*, 83–92. [CrossRef]
16. Green, I.C.; Perrin, D.; Pedley, K.C.; Leslie, R.D.; Pyke, D.A. Effect of enkephalins and morphine on insulin secretion from isolated rat islets. *Diabetologia* **1980**, *19*, 158–161. [CrossRef]
17. Schleicher, R.L. Beta-endorphin inhibits insulin secretion from isolated pancreatic islets. *Endocrinology* **1989**, *124*, 1254–1258. [CrossRef]
18. Czyzyk, T.A.; Romero-Picó, A.; Pintar, J.; McKinzie, J.H.; Tschöp, M.H.; Statnick, M.A.; Nogueiras, R. Mice lacking δ-opioid receptors resist the development of diet-induced obesity. *Faseb. J.* **2012**, *26*, 3483–3492. [CrossRef]
19. Brestoff, J.R.; Kim, B.S.; Saenz, S.A.; Stine, R.R.; Monticelli, L.A.; Sonnenberg, G.F.; Thome, J.J.; Farber, D.L.; Lutfy, K.; Seale, P.; et al. Group 2 innate lymphoid cells promote beiging of white adipose tissue and limit obesity. *Nature* **2015**, *519*, 242–246. [CrossRef]
20. Konig, M.; Zimmer, A.M.; Steiner, H.; Holmes, P.V.; Crawley, J.N.; Brownstein, M.J.; Zimmer, A. Pain responses, anxiety and aggression in mice deficient in pre-proenkephalin. *Nature* **1996**, *383*, 535–538. [CrossRef]
21. Marquez, P.; Baliram, R.; Gajawada, N.; Friedman, T.C.; Lutfy, K. Differential involvement of enkephalins in analgesic tolerance, locomotor sensitization, and conditioned place preference induced by morphine. *Behav. Neurosci.* **2006**, *120*, 10–15. [CrossRef]
22. Tseng, A.; Nguyen, K.; Hamid, A.; Garg, M.; Marquez, P.; Lutfy, K. The role of endogenous beta-endorphin and enkephalins in ethanol reward. *Neuropharmacology* **2013**, *73*, 290–300. [CrossRef]
23. Liu, Y.; Nakagawa, Y.; Wang, Y.; Liu, L.; Du, H.; Wang, W.; Ren, X.; Lutfy, K.; Friedman, T.C. Reduction of hepatic glucocorticoid receptor and hexose-6-phosphate dehydrogenase expression ameliorates diet-induced obesity and insulin resistance in mice. *J. Mol. Endocrinol.* **2008**, *41*, 53–64. [CrossRef]

24. Murray, S.; Tulloch, A.; Gold, M.S.; Avena, N.M. Hormonal and neural mechanisms of food reward, eating behaviour and obesity. *Nat. Rev. Endocrinol.* **2014**, *10*, 540–552. [CrossRef]
25. Richard, D. Cognitive and autonomic determinants of energy homeostasis in obesity. *Nat. Rev. Endocrinol.* **2015**, *11*, 489–501. [CrossRef]
26. Czyzyk, T.A.; Nogueiras, R.; Lockwood, J.F.; McKinzie, J.H.; Coskun, T.; Pintar, J.E.; Hammond, C.; Tschöp, M.H.; Statnick, M.A. kappa-Opioid receptors control the metabolic response to a high-energy diet in mice. *Faseb. J.* **2010**, *24*, 1151–1159. [CrossRef]
27. Tabarin, A.; Diz-Chaves, Y.; Carmona Mdel, C.; Catargi, B.; Zorrilla, E.P.; Roberts, A.J.; Coscina, D.V.; Rousset, S.; Redonnet, A.; Parker, G.C.; et al. Resistance to diet-induced obesity in mu-opioid receptor-deficient mice: Evidence for a "thrifty gene". *Diabetes* **2005**, *54*, 3510–3516. [CrossRef]
28. Wen, T.; Peng, B.; Pintar, J.E. The MOR-1 opioid receptor regulates glucose homeostasis by modulating insulin secretion. *Mol. Endocrinol.* **2009**, *23*, 671–678. [CrossRef]
29. Winzell, M.S.; Ahrén, B. The high-fat diet-fed mouse: A model for studying mechanisms and treatment of impaired glucose tolerance and type 2 diabetes. *Diabetes* **2004**, *53* (Suppl. S3), S215–S219. [CrossRef]
30. Andrikopoulos, S.; Blair, A.R.; Deluca, N.; Fam, B.C.; Proietto, J. Evaluating the glucose tolerance test in mice. *Am J. Physiol. Endocrinol. Metab.* **2008**, *295*, E1323–E1332. [CrossRef]
31. Hatting, M.; Tavares, C.D.J.; Sharabi, K.; Rines, A.K.; Puigserver, P. Insulin regulation of gluconeogenesis. *Ann. N. Y. Acad. Sci.* **2018**, *1411*, 21–35. [CrossRef]

biomedicines

MDPI

Article

Clinical and Pharmacotherapeutic Profile of Patients with Type 2 Diabetes Mellitus Admitted to a Hospital Emergency Department

António Cabral Lopes [1,2,*], Olga Lourenço [2,3], Fátima Roque [3,4] and Manuel Morgado [2,3,4,5]

1 Pharmaceutical Services of Unity Local of Health of Guarda (ULS da Guarda), 6300-035 Guarda, Portugal
2 Health Sciences Faculty, University of Beira Interior (FCS-UBI), 6200-506 Covilhã, Portugal
3 Health Sciences Research Centre, University of Beira Interior (CICS-UBI), 6200-506 Covilhã, Portugal
4 Research Unit for Inland Development, Polytechnic Institute of Guarda (UDI-IPG), 6300-559 Guarda, Portugal
5 Pharmaceutical Services of University Hospital Center of Cova da Beira, 6200-251 Covilhã, Portugal
* Correspondence: antonio.clopes@ulsguarda.min-saude.pt

Abstract: Type 2 diabetes mellitus (T2DM) is closely associated with other pathologies, which may require complex therapeutic approaches. We aim to characterize the clinical and pharmacological profile of T2DM patients admitted to an emergency department. Patients aged ≥65 years and who were already using at least one antidiabetic drug were included in this analysis. Blood glycemia, creatinine, aspartate aminotransferase (AST), alanine aminotransferase (ALT), and hemoglobin were analyzed for each patient, as well as personal pathological history, diagnosis(s) at admission, and antidiabetic drugs used before. Outcome variables were analyzed using Pearson's Chi-Square, Fisher's exact test, and linear regression test. In total, 420 patients were randomly selected (48.6% male and 51.4% female). Patients with family support showed a lower incidence of high glycemia at admission ($p = 0.016$). Higher blood creatinine levels were associated with higher blood glycemia ($p = 0.005$), and hyperuricemia (HU) ($p = 0.001$), as well as HU, was associated with a higher incidence of acute cardiovascular diseases (ACD) ($p = 0.007$). Hemoglobin levels are lower with age ($p = 0.0001$), creatinine ($p = 0.009$), and female gender ($p = 0.03$). The lower the AST/ALT ratio, the higher the glycemia at admission ($p < 0.0001$). Obese patients with ($p = 0.021$) or without ($p = 0.027$) concomitant dyslipidemia had a higher incidence of ACD. Insulin ($p = 0.003$) and glucagon-like peptide-1 agonists (GLP1 RA) ($p = 0.023$) were associated with a higher incidence of decompensated heart failure, while sulfonylureas ($p = 0.009$), metformin-associated with dipeptidyl peptidase-4 inhibitors (DPP4i) ($p = 0.029$) or to a sulfonylurea ($p = 0.003$) with a lower incidence. Metformin, in monotherapy or associated with DPP4i, was associated with a lower incidence of acute kidney injury ($p = 0.017$) or acute chronic kidney injury ($p = 0.014$). SGLT2i monotherapy ($p = 0.0003$), associated with metformin ($p = 0.026$) or with DPP4i ($p = 0.007$), as well as insulin and sulfonylurea association ($p = 0.026$), were associated with hydroelectrolytic disorders, unlike GLP1 RA ($p = 0.017$), DPP4i associated with insulin ($p = 0.034$) or with a GLP1 RA ($p = 0.003$). Insulin was mainly used by autonomous and institutionalized patients ($p = 0.0008$), while metformin ($p = 0.003$) and GLP1 RA ($p < 0.0001$) were used by autonomous patients. Sulfonylureas were mostly used by male patients ($p = 0.027$), while SGLT2 ($p = 0.0004$) and GLP1 RA ($p < 0.0001$) were mostly used by patients within the age group 65-85 years. Sulfonylureas ($p = 0.008$), insulin associated with metformin ($p = 0.040$) or with a sulfonylurea ($p = 0.048$), as well as DPP4i and sulfonylurea association ($p = 0.031$), were associated with higher blood glycemia. T2DM patients are characterized by great heterogeneity from a clinical point of view presenting with several associated comorbidities, so the pharmacotherapeutic approach must consider all aspects that may affect disease progression.

Keywords: Type 2 diabetes mellitus; glycemia; cardiovascular disorders; kidney function

1. Introduction

Diabetes mellitus (DM) is a common condition affecting about 483 million people worldwide and the total number of adults (20–79 years) with the disease in 2045 is estimated to increase to 629 million [1]. If left untreated, DM can cause other life-threatening conditions such as cardiovascular diseases, stroke, chronic kidney disease (CKD), foot ulcers, eye damage, and neuropathy. To date, there is no permanent cure for DM, and patients need to ensure a healthy lifestyle and comply with the pharmacological therapy that best suits their condition [2]. Patients with DM, especially those who are older (≥65), have a lower socioeconomic status, lower health literacy, and do not have familiar or institutional support, are often admitted to hospital emergency services either due to poor glycemic control or to the lack of control of other comorbidities that are closely related. Health professionals must coordinate their intervention to improve glycemic control while maintaining safety, contributing to the improvement of long-term clinical outcomes, and ensuring the sustainability of national healthcare systems [3–5].

Type II diabetes mellitus (T2DM) is the most prevalent form of DM (90%), and it is mainly caused by the combination of two factors: peripheral tissue resistance to insulin and insufficient insulin secretion by pancreatic β cells [6,7]. The increase in the prevalence of T2DM has been mainly driven by rapid urbanization, changes in lifestyle, and poor dietary patterns [8,9]. Several risk factors have been identified for T2DM, such as hyperuricemia, sleep disorders, smoking, depression, cardiovascular disease, dyslipidemia, high blood pressure, aging, ethnicity, family history, physical inactivity, and obesity [10–15].

The provision of health care in this area has evolved over the last few decades, either in the growing specialization of health professionals, increasingly integrated into multidisciplinary teams, or in the emergence of new antidiabetic drugs. These new drugs have allowed not only better glycemic control but also demonstrated protective effects in other concomitant pathologies that greatly contribute to the increase in morbidity and mortality rates in T2DM [16,17]. On the other hand, antidiabetic drugs are increasingly being studied due to the adverse effects that may result from their use, namely their impact on cardiorenal function and electrolytic balance [18,19]. Sodium-glucose co-transporter-2 inhibitors (SGLT2i), Dipeptidyl peptidase-4 inhibitors (DPP4i), and Glucagon-like peptide-1 agonists (GLP1 AR), in addition to hypoglycemic effect, have demonstrated cardiorenal protective effects, while SCLTi has been associated with hydroelectrolytic disorders [20,21].

Insulin, metformin, and sulfonylureas are some of the classic drug classes used to treat T2DM. More recently, new therapeutic approaches have emerged, such as SGLT2i, which increases urinary glucose elimination and blocks its renal absorption; GLP1 AR, which increases insulin secretion by reducing glucagon secretion, delays gastric emptying and promotes satiety; and DPP4i, which inhibits incretin degradation promoting increased insulin secretion and reduced glucagon secretions [22–24].

This work aims to characterize the clinical and pharmacological profile of patients with T2DM who were admitted to the emergency department of the Local Health Unit of Guarda (LHUG), identifying how their clinical condition, on admission time, can be influenced by pre-existing comorbidities and by antidiabetic drugs previously used.

2. Materials and Methods

2.1. Study Design and Sample

A retrospective study of 420 patients with T2DM admitted to the LHUG emergency department from June 2019 to September 2022 was performed. Ethics Committee of the LHUG, Emergency, and Internal Medicine Departments Director's authorizations were obtained.

About 140 patients are admitted to the LHUG emergency department per day, of which about 60% have a known diagnosis of T2DM. Our study includes 39 months of analysis, which amounts to approximately 163,800 admissions episodes in that period (approximately 98,280 patients with a previously known diagnosis of T2DM). This means

383 or more measurements are needed to have a confidence level of 95% that the real value is within ±5% of the measured value.

Patients with the following characteristics were randomly selected (Figure 1):

✓ Diagnosis of T2DM before admission to the emergency department;
✓ At least 65 years of age;
✓ At least one antidiabetic drug included in the chronic treatment plan before admission;
✓ Complete and objective information described in the clinical diary regarding chronic medication, clinical history, and reason(s) for admission to the Emergency Department;
✓ Complete information regarding the analytical parameters included in the study upon admission;
✓ After applying these criteria, a sample of 613 patients was obtained, from which 420 were randomly selected.

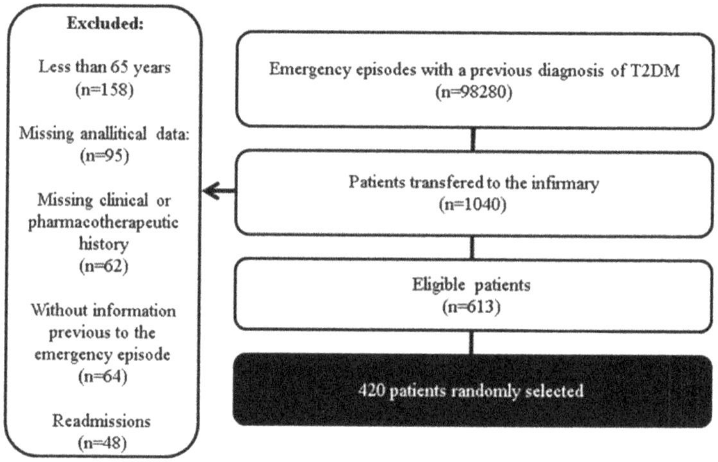

Figure 1. Sample selection.

2.2. Data Collection

Data on patients with T2DM were obtained from the SClinico® and Modulab® platforms. The following variables were analyzed:

✓ Age, gender, and condition (autonomous, family support, or institutionalized);
✓ Bioanalytical parameters at admission: blood glycemia; creatinine; hemoglobin; aspartate aminotransferase (AST), and alanine aminotransferase (ALT);
✓ Personal pathological history: T2DM; high blood pressure (HBP); heart failure (HF); atrial fibrillation (AF); acute myocardial infarction (AMI); dyslipidemia; chronic kidney disease (CKD); hyperuricemia (HU); stroke, obesity; chronic liver disease (CLD); oncological disease (OD); chronic obstructive pulmonary disease (COPD); alcoholism; chronic anemia (CA);
✓ Diagnosis that justifies admission: decompensated heart failure (DHF); acute chronic kidney disease (ACKD); acute kidney injury (AKI); urinary tract infection (UTI); pulmonary embolism (PE); stroke; AMI; respiratory tract infection (RTI); hydroelectrolytic disorders (HED); bleeding; gastroenteritis; acute chronic liver disease (ACLD); pancreatitis; hypoglycemia; respiratory failure; sepsis;
✓ Antidiabetic drugs included in the therapeutic plan before admission: insulin; SGLT2i; DPP4i; GLP1 RA; metformin and sulfonylureas.

2.3. Statistical Analysis

For the statistical analysis, IBM SPSS statistics 28 (IBM, Armonk, NY, USA) was used. Categorical variables were described through their respective absolute and relative frequencies (percentages). Pearson's Chi-Square, Fisher's exact test, and linear regression tests were used with a statistical significance level of 5% ($p < 0.05$).

3. Results

3.1. Sample Characterization

The variables were analyzed in order to verify possible relationships between patients' characteristics (condition, gender, age, laboratory parameters, pathological and pharmacological history) admitted to the emergency department and diagnosis at admission (Table 1).

Table 1. Patients' characteristics at admission.

		Age			
Mean	**80.59**	**Standard Deviation**	**7.92**	**Min-Max**	**65–99**
			Gender		
			Male (n = 204)		**Female (n = 216)**
Autonomous			94 (22.4%)		61 (14.5%)
Family support			49 (11.7%)		42 (10.0%)
Institutionalized			61 (14.5%)		113 (26.9%)
		Pathological history previous to admission			
Type 2 Diabetes Mellitus			204 (48.6%)		216 (51.4%)
High blood pressure			173 (41.2%)		181 (43.1%)
Heart failure			77 (18.3%)		98 (23.3%)
Atrial fibrillation			38 (9.0%)		45 (10.7%)
Acute myocardial infarction			14 (3.3%)		17 (4.0%)
Dyslipidemia			82 (19.5%)		98 (23.3%)
Chronic kidney disease			65 (15.5%)		91 (21.7%)
Hyperuricemia			30 (7.1%)		42 (10.0%)
Stroke			35 (8.3%)		39 (9.3%)
Obesity			27 (6.4%)		44 (10.5%)
Chronic liver disease			17 (4.0%)		6 (1.4%)
Oncological disease			25 (6.0%)		11 (2.6%)
Chronic obstructive pulmonary disease			19 (4.5%)		17 (4.0%)
		Diagnosis at admission			
Decompensated heart failure			43 (10.2%)		66 (15.7%)
Acute chronic kidney disease			46 (11.0%)		67 (16.0%)
Acute kidney injury			66 (15.7%)		51 (12.1%)
Urinary tract infection			14 (3.3%)		28 (6.7%)
Pulmonary embolism			12 (2.9%)		9 (2.1%)
Stroke			18 (4.3%)		19 (4.5%)
Acute myocardial infarction			9 (2.1%)		8 (1.9%)
Respiratory tract infection			56 (12.9%)		65 (15.5%)
Hydroelectrolytic disorders			94 (22.4%)		92 (21.9%)
Bleeding			3 (0.7%)		0 (0.0%)
Gastroenteritis			4 (1.0%)		2 (0.5%)
Acute chronic liver disease			12 (2.9%)		5 (1.2%)
Pancreatitis			3 (0.7%)		3 (0.7%)
Hypoglycemia			2 (0.5%)		2 (0.5%)
Respiratory failure			59 (14.0%)		74 (17.6%)
Sepsis			5 (1.2%)		11 (2.6%)

Table 1. *Cont.*

Age					
Mean	**80.59**	**Standard Deviation**	**7.92**	**Min-Max**	**65–99**
			Gender		
			Male (n = 204)		**Female (n = 216)**
Antidiabetic drugs included in the therapeutic plan before admission					
Insulin			100 (23.8%)		127 (30.2%)
Sodium-glucose cotransporter inhibitors			54 (12.9%)		54 (12.9%)
Dipeptidyl peptidase inhibitors			111 (26.4%)		107 (25.5%)
Glucagon-like peptide-1 receptor agonists			10 (2.4%)		17 (4.0%)
Metformin			107 (25.5%)		96 (22.9%)
Sulfonylureas			36 (8.6%)		22 (5.2%)
Laboratory parameters at admission					
Glycemia			Blood creatinine		
<180 mg/dL		≥180 mg/dL	<1.2 mg/dL		≥1.2 mg/dL
183 (43.6%)		237 (56.4%)	170 (40.5%)		250 (59.5%)

The American Diabetes Association classifies glycemia above 180 mg/dL as hyperglycemia; therefore, patients were classified according to this reference value [25].

A cut-off value of 1.2 mg/dL was considered for blood creatinine (for men with normal kidney function is approximately 0.6 to 1.2mg/dL and between 0.5 to 1.1 mg/dL for women) [26].

3.2. Relationship between Patient's Condition before Admission, Age, and Gender with Glycemia Levels

There was a statistically significant association between the patient's condition and glycemia levels at admission (p = 0.016, Pearson's Chi-Square). Patients with family support showed a lower incidence of hyperglycemia (9.5%) than autonomous (23.1%) and institutionalized (23.8%) (Table 2). On the other hand, there was no statistically significant association between gender and glycemia levels (p = 0.862, Pearson's Chi-Square), as well as between age and glycemia levels at admission (p = 0.281, Pearson's Chi-Square).

Table 2. Relationship between patient's condition, gender, and age with glycemia levels.

	Condition				
Glycemia	**Autonomous**	**Family Support**	**Institutionalized**	**Total**	***p*-Value**
<180 mg/dL	58 (13.8%)	51 (12.1%)	74 (7.6%)	183 (43.6%)	0.016 *
≥180 mg/dL	97 (23.1%)	40 (9.5%)	100 (23.8%)	237 (56.4%)	
Total	155 (36.9%)	91 (21.7%)	174 (41.4%)	420 (100%)	

* Pearson's Chi-Square.

3.3. Hyperuricemia, Hemoglobin, and AST/ALT Ratio

3.3.1. Hyperuricemia

According to our results, there was a statistically significant association between blood creatinine levels and glycemia (p = 0.005, Pearson's Chi-Square) and HU (p = 0.001, Pearson's Chi-Square). Patients with blood glycemia levels above 180 mg/dL and a history of HU had higher blood creatinine values (≥1.2 mg/dL) at admission. There was also a statistically significant association between HU and acute CVD (decompensated heart failure, stroke, acute myocardial infarction, and/or pulmonary embolism) at admission (p = 0.007, Pearson's Chi-Square).

3.3.2. Hemoglobin and T2DM

In order to relate hemoglobin levels at admission to gender, age, and blood creatinine (<1.2 mg/dL or ≥1.2 mg/dL), we used a linear regression model using the ("stepwise" method). It was observed that the variables age (p = 0.0001), creatinine (p = 0.001), and gender ($p = 0.03$) were significant in the model. The regression equation obtained (Hb = 17.130–0.056 (Age)—0.766 (Creatinine above 1.2 mg/dL)—0.492 (Gender)) indicates that hemoglobin values decrease with age, being lower in female patients and with creatinine values above 1.2 mg/dL.

3.3.3. AST/ALT Ratio

The relationship between glycemia (converted to the Neperian logarithm) and the AST/ALT ratio was analyzed through a linear regression model. According to the regression equation (Ln(Glycemia)) = 5.503–0.159 (AST/ALT ratio), the lower the AST/ALT ratio, the higher the glycemia levels at admission ($p < 0.0001$).

3.4. Obesity, Dyslipidemia, and Acute Cardiovascular Disorders

Obese patients with or without concomitant dyslipidemia (Table 1) were exposed to a higher risk of acute cardiovascular disorders (DHF, AMI, Stroke, and/or PE) at admission (OR 2.049, 95% CI 1.075–3.906, $p = 0.027$, Pearson's Chi-Square) and (OR 1.825, 95% CI 1.092–3.051, $p = 0.021$, Pearson's Chi-Square), respectively than non-obese patients.

3.5. Antidiabetic Therapy and Heart Failure

Our findings suggest that patients using insulin ($p = 0.003$), GLP1 RA ($p = 0.023$) or both associated ($p = 0.007$) were exposed to a higher risk of DHF at admission, while patients using sulfonylureas ($p = 0.009$), metformin and DPP4i association ($p = 0.029$) and metformin and sulfonylurea association ($p = 0.003$) to a lower risk (Table 3).

Table 3. Relationship between decompensated heart failure and antidiabetic therapy.

Previously Diagnosed Heart Failure			Decompensated Heart Failure at Admission		
Yes 175 (41.7%)	No 245 (58.3%)		Yes 109 (26.0%)	No 311 (74.0%)	
Antidiabetic Drugs	**Decompensated HF (No/Yes)**		***p*-Value**	**OR**	**Confidence Interval 95%**
Insulin	155 (49.8%)	72 (66.1%)	$p = 0.003$ *	1.959	1.243–3.085
GLP1 RA	15 (4.8%)	12 (11.0%)	$p = 0.023$ *	2.441	1.105–5.395
Sulfonylureas	51 (16.4%)	7 (6.4%)	$p = 0.009$ *	0.350	0.154–0.796
Insulin + GLP1 RA	9 (2.9%)	10 (9.2%)	$p = 0.007$ *	3.389	1.339–8.579
Metformin + DPP4i	100 (32.2%)	23 (21.1%)	$p = 0.029$ *	0.564	0.336–0.947
Metformin + Sulfonylurea	38 (12.2%)	3 (2.8%)	$p = 0.003$ **	0.203	0.061–0.673

* Pearson's Chi-Square. ** Fisher's exact test.

3.6. Antidiabetic Therapy and Kidney Function

Patients undergoing treatment with metformin ($p = 0.017$) or metformin and DPP4i association ($p = 0.014$) were exposed to a lower risk of AKI or ACKD (Table 4).

Patients using SGLT2i ($p = 0.0003$), insulin and sulfonylurea association ($p = 0.026$), metformin and SGLT2i association (OR $p = 0.026$), and DPP4i and SGLT2i association ($p = 0.007$) were exposed to a higher risk of hydroelectrolytic disorders. On the other hand, patients using GLP1 RA ($p = 0.017$), insulin and DPP4i association ($p = 0.034$), or DPP4i and GLP1 RA association ($p = 0.003$) had a lower risk of hydroelectrolytic disorders (Table 4).

Table 4. Relationship between antidiabetic therapy and acute kidney injury, acute chronic kidney injury, and hydroelectrolytic disorders.

Antidiabetic Drugs	AKI or ACKD (n = 230)	*p*-Value	OR	Confidence Interval 95%
Metformin	99 (43.0%)	0.017 *	0.625	0.424–0.920
Metformin + DPP4i	56 (24.3%)	0.014 *	0.521	0.387–0.902
	Hydroelectrolytic disorders			
SGLT2i	64 (34.4%)	0.0003 *	2.265	1.450–3.539
GLP1 RA	6 (3.2%)	0.017 *	0.338	0.134–0.856
Insulin + DPP4i	38 (20.4%)	0.034 *	0.614	0.390–0.967
Insulin + Sulfonylurea	8 (4.3%)	0.026 **	5.213	1.094–24.853
Metformin + SGLT2i	34 (18.3%)	0.026 *	1.870	1.071–3.264
DPP4i + SGLT2i	29 (15.6%)	0.007 *	2.358	1.252–4.440
DPP4i + GLP1 RA	0 (0.0%)	0.003 **	0.957	0.932–0.984

* Pearson's Chi-Square. ** Fisher's exact test.

3.7. *Antidiabetic Therapy and Glycemia Levels*

Our findings suggest that insulin is mainly used by autonomous and institutionalized patients ($p = 0.0008$, Pearson's Chi-Square), while metformin ($p = 0.003$, Pearson's Chi-Square) and GLP1 RA ($p = 4 \times 10^{-6}$, Fisher's exact test) are mainly used by autonomous patients. On the other hand, Sulphonylureas are mostly used by male patients ($p = 0.027$, Pearson's Chi-Square), while SGLT2 ($p = 0.0004$, Pearson's Chi-Square) and GLP1 RA ($p < 0.0001$, Pearson's Chi-Square) are mostly used by patients within the age group 65–85 years. Patients treated with sulfonylureas ($p = 0.008$), insulin and metformin association ($p = 0.040$), insulin and sulfonylurea association ($p = 0.048$), and DPP4i and sulfonylurea association ($p = 0.031$) were exposed to a higher risk of hyperglycemia (≥180 mg/dL) at admission (Table 5).

Table 5. Relationship between Antidiabetic drugs and serum glycemia level at admission.

Antidiabetic Drugs	Glycemia ≥ 180 mg/dL (No/Yes)		*p*-Value	OR	Confidence Interval 95%
Sulfonylureas	16 (8.7%)	42 (17.7%)	$p = 0.008$ *	2.248	1.219–4.145
Insulin + Metformin	20 (10.9%)	43 (18.1%)	$p = 0.040$ *	1.806	1.022–3.194
Insulin + Sulfonylurea	1 (0.5%)	9 (3.8%)	$p = 0.048$ **	7.184	0.902–57.227
DPP4i + Sulfonylurea	11 (6.0%)	29 (12.2%)	$p = 0.031$ *	4.644	1.058–4.492

* Pearson's Chi-Square. ** Fisher's exact test.

4. Discussion

4.1. *Glycemia Levels and Patients' Characteristics*

Glycemic control in patients with T2DM is influenced by the type of family and social support they may have [27,28]. It is extremely important to include the patient, their family, and caretakers in the clinical decisions to achieve adherence to T2DM self-management, especially because much of the process takes place within the family environment [29]. Our findings suggest that patients with T2DM and good family support had better glycemic control upon admission to the emergency department compared to autonomous or institutionalized patients (Table 2). These results are in line with other studies in this field, according to which T2DM self-management education with family support improves health outcomes for patients with uncontrolled glycemia [30,31].

4.2. *Impact of Hyperuricemia on Kidney Function and Cardiovascular System*

HU is a condition that appears to be associated with increased insulin resistance and the onset and progression of diabetic complications [32]. Evidence provided by epidemiological studies suggests that HU is also a risk factor for HBP, CKD, and cardiovascular disease (CVD) [33]. HU in patients with T2DM is an important risk factor for both cardiovascular disease and kidney function deterioration [34–37]. An elevated uric acid level is a marker of cardiovascular risk. However, this association is not independent of some indicators of kidney function impairment, such as albuminuria or decreased glomerular filtration rate [38]. Several observational studies have identified HU as a risk factor for the development and/or progression of kidney disease, with some clinical trials suggesting that reducing uric acid levels with allopurinol could have beneficial effects in preventing or delaying kidney function deterioration [39]. However, recent studies have failed to statistically demonstrate the benefit of allopurinol on kidney function in these circumstances [40,41]. A likely explanation for the discrepancy between these studies and previous observational studies is that the predictive effect of HU on the loss of kidney function may be indirect and attributable to its association with other causally related features of kidney disease, such as insulin resistance and metabolic syndrome [42]. Regarding the potential effects of antidiabetic therapy in this domain, a recent study suggests that SGLT2i have an anti-inflammatory activity via uric acid and insulin by reducing the respective levels, with cardiovascular and renal benefits [43].

Our findings suggest that patients with HU had a higher incidence of acute cardiovascular disorders at admission. Moreover, patients with HU and higher glycemia levels ($\geq$180 mg/dL) had higher levels of serum creatinine and urea and, therefore, greater worsening of kidney function, in line with what has been reported in other studies.

4.3. Relationship between Hemoglobin Levels, Gender, Age, and Kidney Function

Patients with T2DM are more susceptible to the development of chronic anemia, which may be due to inadequate glycemic control, CKD (that leads to erythropoietin production decrease), presence of T2DM complications, or age >60 years [44–46]. Previous studies have shown that diabetic females and diabetic elderly are the most vulnerable groups to anemia; moreover, having high blood creatinine is an important influence at this level [47,48]. According to our findings, female gender, older age, and serum creatinine values above 1.2 mg/dL, are related to lower hemoglobin levels.

4.4. Liver Function and Serum Glycemia Levels

Both AST and ALT have metabolic functions and are expressed in multiple organs, including the liver, myocardium, and skeletal muscle. ALT is mainly expressed in the liver, while AST is widely expressed, including in skeletal muscle. Therefore, a high serum ALT activity reflects the destruction of hepatocytes, while a high serum AST activity, along with a normal ALT activity, may reflect muscle damage [49,50]. Patients with T2DM have a higher incidence of liver functions tests showing abnormalities than individuals who do not have the disease. In addition, non-alcoholic fatty liver disease is very prevalent [51]. An increasing AST/ALT ratio is associated with declining glucose regulation, metabolic impairment, and organ dysfunction, including non-alcoholic fatty liver disease and cardiovascular disease [52]. Some recent studies reported that AST/ALT ratio increases is inversely related to metabolic syndrome development. It is accepted that an AST/ALT ratio is inversely associated with T2DM occurrence [53]. Our findings suggest that higher glycemia values at admission are associated with a lower AST/ALT ratio.

4.5. Patients' Pharmacotherapeutic Profile and Acute Cardiovascular Disease

There is a close link between T2DM and cardiovascular diseases, which are the most prevalent cause of morbidity and mortality in diabetic patients [54,55]. Cardiovascular risk factors such as obesity, hypertension, and dyslipidemia are common in patients with T2DM, putting them at an increased risk for cardiovascular events [56,57]. T2DM is an important risk factor for the development of micro and macrovascular complications, including coronary artery disease, AKI, ACKD, and even stroke [58]. In patients with T2DM, glycated hemoglobin (HbA1c) level $\geq$ 7.0% was the strongest predictor of stroke and acute myocardial infarction [59]. Epidemiological studies have shown that a 1% increase in HbA1c levels leads to a 15 to 18% increase in cardiovascular events in patients with T2DM [60]. Intensive glycemic control aims to obtain an HbA1C of less than 7%, contributing to the prevention or the progression delay of microvascular complications, such as diabetic retinopathy and CKD, in patients with T2DM [24]. In contrast, the available information on the association between glycemic control and macrovascular diseases is limited since the glycemic control profiles of antidiabetic drugs in various cardiovascular complications have not yet been clearly elucidated [61,62]. Our findings indicate that obese patients, with or without concomitant dyslipidemia, showed a higher incidence of cardiovascular adverse events.

The recent realization that several antidiabetic drug classes approved may have divergent effects on HF and that some classes of agents may reduce the risk of HF has triggered different studies to establish a more predictable relationship between treatments and outcomes [63,64]. Some cardiovascular controlled trials have demonstrated the ability of iSGLT2 to reduce major cardiovascular adverse events and hospitalization for heart failure [65–67]. Dapagliflozin was even recently approved in Europe for the treatment of HF with reduced ejection fraction [68]. A recent study showed that metformin utilization compared to sulfonylureas in T2DM patients with worsening renal function was associated with reduced hospitalization for HF [69]. Although, recent large randomized controlled trials have not shown differences in cardiovascular risk of sulfonylureas versus pioglitazone or linagliptin [70]. Some studies point to a higher incidence of DHF in patients with T2DM taking sulfonylureas; others show inconclusive data [71].

Our findings demonstrated that patients using sulfonylureas, metformin, and iDPP4 association and metformin and sulfonylurea association were exposed to a lower risk of DHF. On the other hand, our findings did not show any benefit of SGLTi in this parameter (Table 3).

4.6. Patients' Pharmacotherapeutic Profile and Kidney Disease

The pathophysiology of kidney disease in T2DM is characterized by multifactorial critical impairment. Hyperglycemic states lead to dysregulated intracellular metabolism, inflammatory kidney damage, increased apoptosis processes, and tissue fibrosis [72]. Higher HbA1c was associated with AKI in adults with T2DM and CKD, suggesting that improving glycemic control may reduce the risk of AKI [73]. The impact of antidiabetic drugs on renal function is increasingly studied. Dapagliflozin (SGLTi), for example, has been shown to be able to reduce the incidence of renal events and to prolong CKD patients' survival, with and without T2DM [74].

Our findings demonstrated that patients undergoing treatment with metformin or metformin and DPP4i association were exposed to a lower risk of AKI or ACKD, revealing a protective effect (Table 4). Current experimental and clinical data provide some evidence for metformin as a promising pharmacological tool for renal diseases with or without T2DM [75]. Based on experimental evidence and some relevant clinical observations, metformin seems to be a promising drug in the treatment of progressive renal damage [76].

Antidiabetic drugs are associated with certain acid-base and HED, which should be taken into account in the decision process of T2DM treatment [77]. Our findings suggest that patients taking iSGLT2, insulin and sulfonylurea association, metformin and iSGLT2 association or iDPP4 and iSGLT2 were exposed to a higher risk of hydroelectrolytic disorders, unlike patients using ARGLP1, insulin, and iDPP4 association or iDPP4 and ARGLP1 association, that were exposed to a lower risk in this domain (Table 4). Although clinical data suggest that iSGLT2s are safe and protect against renal and cardiovascular events, little attention has been devoted to the effects of these compounds in the renal treatment of different electrolytes. Although a natriuretic effect and osmotic diuresis are expected, these compounds may also modulate the urinary excretion of potassium, magnesium, phosphate, and calcium. Some of the disturbances of homeostasis are transient, while others may persist, suggesting that the administration of these compounds may induce new electrolyte homeostasis [78].

4.7. Relationship between Patients' Profile and Anti-Diabetic Drugs Used

According to our findings, metformin is more commonly used by autonomous patients (Table 5). This may arise because it is the recommended first-line treatment in T2DM and is used in earlier stages of the disease when most patients do not need any kind of support (familiar or institutional) [79]. Insulin is mostly used by autonomous and institutionalized patients because it is a therapeutic option that requires more controlled administration management [80]. GLP1 RA is mostly used by autonomous and younger patients. This fact may be due to its indication in obese patients and, therefore, in the reduction in the risks associated with this comorbidity. Furthermore, its subcutaneous administration also presupposes some autonomy or some type of support [81]. Sulphonylureas are used more by male than female patients. This comes in line with previous studies, according to which male gender and lower body mass indices are associated with a better glycemic response with sulfonylureas [82]. SGLT2i are mostly used by patients within the age group 65–85 years compared to older patients. In general, they are well tolerated; however, some caution is recommended in older patients who use other concomitant therapies such as diuretics [83].

4.8. Relationship between Glycemic Levels at Admission and Antidiabetic Drugs

The impact of antidiabetic drugs on glycemic control in the real world does not always match the results reported in clinical trials. In addition, non-adherence to therapy may be influenced by patient-centered and therapy-related factors [84–87]. According to some previous studies, the pattern of antidiabetic drugs' use varies between different age groups and gender. Metformin, for example, due to its low risk for hypoglycemia, may be beneficial in older adults, and its low cost may make it an efficient choice [88,89]. On the other hand, factors related to therapy, including medication route, treatment duration, treatment complexity (a fixed-dose combination can lead to a significant improvement in adherence to pharmacological therapy of T2DM compared to a loose-dose combination), drug type, and drug side effects, are aspects that also influence the pattern of antidiabetic drugs' use [90,91]. In addition, new-generation antidiabetic drugs are less studied than other, more traditional therapeutic options, so their effects, both in terms of efficacy and safety, may be less predictable, particularly in more vulnerable populations, such as the elderly [92]. Dosage adjustments are often required due to factors such as suboptimal medication adherence, psychosocial profiles, lifestyle, and health-seeking behavior [93,94]. Several comparative studies were carried out to assess the effectiveness of different antidiabetic drugs in glycemic control. In general, inadequately-controlled T2DM patients can benefit from using a combination of two or more different antidiabetic drugs [95,96]. If the HbA1C level is greater than 7.5% during treatment or if the baseline HbA1C is $\geq$9%, combination therapy with two oral antidiabetic drugs or with insulin may be considered [25,97]. There has been major progress in T2DM pharmacological treatment during the last few years. The rapid pace at which diabetology is developing makes it challenging to keep up with the interesting and innovative therapeutic approaches currently used [98].

Different recombinant insulin analogs have different mechanisms of action: rapid-acting insulin analogs provide a bolus level of insulin needed with meals (prandial insulin); longer-acting insulins released slowly over a longer period provide the required level of basal insulin throughout the day and night. Although insulin has been an important discovery for the treatment of DM, it is rarely used as a first-line treatment option for T2DM. Insulin administration carries risks of developing severe hypoglycemia and cardiovascular complications and occurs more often when patients develop insulin tolerance and an increase in doses is required [99,100].

Metformin monotherapy lowers fasting plasma glucose and glycated hemoglobin in a first-line approach to the T2DM patient. It is currently the only antihyperglycemic drug recommended by the American Diabetes Association and the European Association for the Study of Diabetes as initial oral therapy for patients with T2DM [101,102].

Sulfonylureas have been widely prescribed to treat T2DM. They are well tolerated, and their popularity can be attributed to their low cost and the possibility of being used as monotherapy or in combination with metformin [103]. Sulphonylureas interact not only with their receptors on pancreatic β-cells but also with smooth muscle cells and cardiac myocytes, which may explain why they are associated with a higher prevalence of hypoglycemia and cardiovascular risk [104,105]. However, most reports support the cardiovascular safety of sulfonylureas [106].

iDPP4s have been shown to be non-inferior to classical antidiabetic drugs and to be well tolerated with almost no side effects or episodes of hypoglycemia, with a neutral or slightly beneficial effect on body weight. Its oral administration and fixed doses without the need for escalation are other characteristics that facilitated adherence to this type of therapy. They are effective in improving glycemic control, mainly when used in association with metformin or other antidiabetic drugs, including insulin. The near absence of side effects and its weight neutrality, in contrast to sulfonylureas, thiazolidinediones, or even insulin, made this class of drugs one of the most used after metformin [107,108].

GLP-1 ARs promote glycemic control through a multitude of widely recognized physiological mechanisms, among them stimulation of insulin secretion and inhibition of glucagon release, directly improving postprandial glucose homeostasis, while inhibition of gastric emptying and food intake represents a long-term positive effect in limiting weight gain. Several cardiovascular outcomes studies have shown that GLP-1 RAs can effectively prevent cardiovascular events such as AMI or stroke and associated mortality. The underlying mechanisms may be related to the inhibition of the progression of atherosclerotic lesions. Therefore, the guidelines particularly recommend GLP-1 RA treatment in patients with pre-existing atherosclerotic vascular disease [109,110].

iSGLT2s binds competitively to glucose transporters reducing its reabsorption by renal tubular epithelial cells, promoting urinary excretion and, consequently, exerting hypoglycemic effects. They have demonstrated good effectiveness in glycemic control in a non-insulin-dependent way [111,112].

Our findings suggest that patients treated with insulin (when associated with metformin or sulfonylurea) and sulfonylureas (with or without DPP4i associated) were exposed to a higher risk of hyperglycemia at admission (Table 5). Some studies demonstrated that patients on insulin were more likely to have poorly controlled glycemia than those on metformin alone [113,114]. Sulphonylureas are generally associated with hypoglycemia risk, particularly in the elderly, which contradicts our findings [115]. Although, most of these patients presented clinical conditions of considerable stress. Stress-induced hyperglycemia is a condition that develops in patients undergoing any form of clinical stress and that occurs due to an increase in peripheral insulin resistance, a decrease in its secretion, and increased glucose production [116]. Sulphonylureas stimulate insulin secretion, metformin decreases glucose synthesis, and endogenous insulin acts on its specific receptors. All these mechanisms are affected by stress-induced hyperglycemia, and a more robust approach to glycemic control and stabilization may be necessary. The treatment consists of intravenous insulin infusion [117].

5. Conclusions

T2DM patients are characterized by great heterogeneity from a clinical point of view. Usually, they have several associated comorbidities, so the pharmacotherapeutic approach must consider all aspects that may affect the progress of the disease. Health professionals should contribute to improving patients' health literacy, as it directly influences management and self-care skills, glycemic control, and patients' quality of life, contributing to better health outcomes.

Our findings corroborate some of the previously established relationships, both in clinical and pharmacological terms, as well as demonstrate that patients have better glycemic control and disease management when they benefit from adequate social and family support. However, some aspects may have influenced our results: this is a monocentric study that includes patients from a restricted geographic area with advanced mean age and several associated comorbidities; most patients have chronic pharmacotherapeutic plans that include different drugs with a wide range of effects and interactions; there is no information available on the stage of diabetic disease in which each patient; most of these patients were in a complex clinical situation at admission.

Author Contributions: O.L., M.M. and F.R. were involved in the conception and design; all authors were involved in the analysis and interpretation of the data; A.C.L. wrote the first draft of the paper and all authors revised it critically for intellectual content and approved the final version to be published; all authors agree to be accountable for all aspects of the work. All authors have read and agreed to the published version of the manuscript.

Funding: This research received no external funding.

Institutional Review Board Statement: The study was conducted in accordance with the Declaration of Helsinki, and approved by the Ethics Committee of the Local Health Unit of Guarda.

Informed Consent Statement: Patient consent was waived due because the ethics committee of the Local Health Unit in Guarda considered that it would be unnecessary in this case.

Data Availability Statement: Not applicable.

Conflicts of Interest: The authors declare no conflict of interest.

References

1. International Diabetes Federation. *IDF Diabetes Atlas*, 10th ed.; International Diabetes Federation: Brussels, Belgium, 2021.
2. Complications of Diabetes. Available online: https://www.mayoclinic.org/diseases-conditions/diabetes/symptoms-causes/syc-20371444 (accessed on 20 November 2022).
3. Curtis, A.J.; Lee, W.A.A. Spatial patterns of diabetes related health problems for vulnerable populations in Los Angeles. *Int. J. Health Geogr.* **2010**, *9*, 43. [CrossRef] [PubMed]
4. Agidew, E.; Wale, M.Z.; Kerebih, H.; Yirsaw, M.T.; Zewdie, T.H.; Girma, M.; Miskir, A. Adherence to diabetes self-care management and associated factors among people with diabetes in Gamo Gofa Zone public health hospitals. *SAGE Open Med.* **2021**, *9*, 20503121211053953. [CrossRef] [PubMed]
5. Souza, J.G.; Farfel, J.M.; Jaluul, O.; Queiroz, M.S.; Nery, M. Association between health literacy and glycemic control in elderly patients with type 2 diabetes and modifying effect of social support. *Einstein* **2020**, *18*, eAO5572. [CrossRef] [PubMed]
6. Roden, M.; Shulman, G.I. The integrative biology of type 2 diabetes. *Nature* **2019**, *576*, 51–60. [CrossRef] [PubMed]
7. Galicia-Garcia, U.; Benito-Vicente, A.; Jebari, S.; Larrea-Sebal, A.; Siddiqi, H.; Uribe, K.B.; Ostolaza, H.; Martín, C. Pathophysiology of Type 2 Diabetes Mellitus. *Int. J. Mol. Sci.* **2020**, *21*, 6275. [CrossRef] [PubMed]
8. Goryakin, Y.; Rocco, L.; Suhrcke, M. The contribution of urbanization to non-communicable diseases: Evidence from 173 countries from 1980 to 2008. *Econ. Hum. Biol.* **2017**, *26*, 151–163. [CrossRef] [PubMed]
9. Hu, F.B. Globalization of diabetes: The role of diet, lifestyle, and genes. *Diabetes Care* **2011**, *34*, 1249–1257. [CrossRef]
10. Alqahtani, S.A.M.; Awan, Z.A.; Alasmary, M.Y.; Al Amoudi, S.M. Association between serum uric acid with diabetes and other biochemical markers. *J. Family Med. Prim. Care* **2022**, *11*, 1401–1409. [CrossRef]
11. Cappuccio, F.P.; D'Elia, L.; Strazzullo, P.; Miller, M.A. Quantity and quality of sleep and incidence of type 2 diabetes: A systematic review and meta-analysis. *Diabetes Care* **2010**, *33*, 414–420. [CrossRef]
12. Maddatu, J.; Anderson-Baucum, E.; Evans-Molina, C. Smoking and the risk of type 2 diabetes. *Transl. Res.* **2017**, *184*, 101–107. [CrossRef]
13. Darwish, L.; Beroncal, E.; Sison, M.V.; Swardfager, W. Depression in people with type 2 diabetes: Current perspectives. *Diabetes Metab. Syndr. Obes.* **2018**, *11*, 333–343. [CrossRef]
14. Qiu, L.; Wang, W.; Sa, R.; Liu, F. Prevalence and Risk Factors of Hypertension, Diabetes, and Dyslipidemia among Adults in Northwest China. *Int. J. Hypertens.* **2021**, *2021*, 5528007. [CrossRef]
15. Cederberg, H.; Stančáková, A.; Kuusisto, J.; Laakso, M.; Smith, U. Family history of type 2 diabetes increases the risk of both obesity and its complications: Is type 2 diabetes a disease of inappropriate lipid storage? *J. Intern. Med.* **2015**, *277*, 540–551. [CrossRef]
16. Nigussie, S.; Birhan, N.; Amare, F.; Mengistu, G.; Adem, F.; Abegaz, T.M. Rate of glycemic control and associated factors among type two diabetes mellitus patients in Ethiopia: A cross sectional study. *PLoS ONE* **2021**, *16*, e0251506. [CrossRef]
17. Cao, H.; Liu, T.; Wang, L.; Ji, Q. Comparative efficacy of novel antidiabetic drugs on cardiovascular and renal outcomes in patients with diabetic kidney disease: A systematic review and network meta-analysis. *Diabetes Obes. Metab.* **2022**, *24*, 1448–1457. [CrossRef]
18. Zanchi, A.; Lehmann, R.; Philippe, J. Antidiabetic drugs and kidney disease–recommendations of the Swiss Society for Endocrinology and Diabetology. *Swiss Med. Wkly.* **2012**, *142*, w13629. [CrossRef]

19. Filippatos, T.; Tzavella, E.; Rizos, C.; Elisaf, M.; Liamis, G. Acid-base and electrolyte disorders associated with the use of antidiabetic drugs. *Expert Opin. Drug. Saf.* **2017**, *16*, 1121–1132. [CrossRef]
20. Giugliano, D.; Longo, M.; Signoriello, S.; Maiorino, M.I.; Solerte, B.; Chiodini, P.; Esposito, K. The effect of DPP-4 inhibitors, GLP-1 receptor agonists and SGLT-2 inhibitors on cardiorenal outcomes: A network meta-analysis of 23 CVOTs. *Cardiovasc. Diabetol.* **2022**, *21*, 42. [CrossRef]
21. Razavi, M.; Wei, Y.Y.; Rao, X.Q.; Zhong, J.X. DPP-4 inhibitors and GLP-1RAs: Cardiovascular safety and benefits. *Military Med. Res.* **2022**, *9*, 45. [CrossRef]
22. Trevor, A.J.; Kruidering-Hall, M.; Katzung, B.G.; Tuan, R.L.; Vanderah, T.W. *Katzung & Trevor's Pharmacology: Examination & Board Review*, 13th ed.; Mc Graw Hill: New York, NY, USA, 2021.
23. Wells, B.; DiPiro, J.; Schwinghammer, T.; Dipiro, C. *Pharmacotherapy Manual*; McGraw Hill Eduaction: New York, NY, USA, 2016.
24. Pape, E.; Nascimento, E.; Jordão, A. *Fármacos na Diabetes*; LIDEL: Lisboa, Portugal, 2019.
25. American Diabetes Association Professional Practice Committee. 6. Glycemic Targets: Standards of Medical Care in Diabetes—2022. *Diabetes Care* **2022**, *45* (Suppl. 1), S83–S96. [CrossRef]
26. Shahbaz, H.; Gupta, M. *Creatinine Clearance*; StatPearls Publishing: Treasure Island, FL, USA, 2022. Available online: http://www.ncbi.nlm.nih.gov/books/NBK544228/ (accessed on 24 October 2022).
27. Olagbemide, O.J.; Omosanya, O.E.; Ayodapo, A.O.; Agboola, S.M.; Adeagbo, A.O.; Olukokun, T.A. Family support and medication adherence among adult type 2 diabetes: Any meeting point? *Ann. Afr. Med.* **2021**, *20*, 282–287. [CrossRef] [PubMed]
28. de Sousa-Munoz, R.L.; de Sá, A.D. Apoio social, funcionalidade familiar e controle glicêmico de pacientes diabéticos tipo 2. *Revista De Medicina* **2020**, *99*, 432–441. [CrossRef]
29. Bennich, B.B.; Røder, M.E.; Overgaard, D.; Egerod, I.; Munch, L.; Knop, F.K.; Vilsbøll, T.; Konradsen, H. Supportive and non-supportive interactions in families with a type 2 diabetes patient: An integrative review. *Diabetol. Metab. Syndr.* **2017**, *9*, 57. [CrossRef] [PubMed]
30. Pamungkas, R.A.; Chamroonsawasdi, K.; Vatanasomboon, P. A Systematic Review: Family Support Integrated with Diabetes Self-Management among Uncontrolled Type II Diabetes Mellitus Patients. *Behav. Sci.* **2017**, *7*, 62. [CrossRef] [PubMed]
31. Gonzalez-Zacarias, A.A.; Mavarez-Martinez, A.; Arias-Morales, C.E.; Stoicea, N.; Rogers, B. Impact of Demographic, Socioeconomic, and Psychological Factors on Glycemic Self-Management in Adults with Type 2 Diabetes Mellitus. *Front. Public Health* **2016**, *4*, 195. [CrossRef] [PubMed]
32. Kushiyama, A.; Tanaka, K.; Hara, S.; Kawazu, S. Linking uric acid metabolism to diabetic complications. *World J. Diabetes* **2014**, *5*, 787–795. [CrossRef]
33. Nishizawa, H.; Maeda, N.; Shimomura, I. Impact of hyperuricemia on chronic kidney disease and atherosclerotic cardiovascular disease. *Hypertens. Res.* **2022**, *45*, 635–640. [CrossRef]
34. Agarwal, A.K.; Singh, M.; Arya, V.; Garg, U.; Singh, V.P.; Jain, V. Prevalence of peripheral arterial disease in type 2 diabetes mellitus and its correlation with coronary artery disease and its risk factors. *J. Assoc. Physicians. India* **2012**, *60*, 28–32.
35. Arersa, K.K.; Wondimnew, T.; Welde, M.; Husen, T.M. Prevalence and Determinants of Hyperuricemia in Type 2 Diabetes Mellitus Patients Attending Jimma Medical Center, Southwestern Ethiopia, 2019. *Diabetes Metab. Syndr. Obes.* **2020**, *13*, 2059–2067. [CrossRef]
36. Li, G.X.; Jiao, X.H.; Cheng, X.B. Correlations between blood uric acid and the incidence and progression of type 2 diabetes nephropathy. *Eur. Rev. Med. Pharmacol. Sci.* **2018**, *22*, 506–511. [CrossRef]
37. Ozsu, S.; Çoşar, A.M.; Aksoy, H.B.; Bülbül, Y.; Oztuna, F.; Karahan, S.C.; Ozlu, T. Prognostic Value of Uric Acid for Pulmonary Thromboembolism. *Respir. Care* **2017**, *62*, 1091–1096. [CrossRef]
38. Kim, H.K.; Lee, M.; Lee, Y.H.; Lee, B.W.; Cha, B.S.; Kang, E.S. Uric Acid Variability as a Predictive Marker of Newly Developed Cardiovascular Events in Type 2 Diabetes. *Front. Cardiovasc. Med.* **2021**, *8*, 775753. [CrossRef]
39. Gherghina, M.E.; Peride, I.; Tiglis, M.; Neagu, T.P.; Niculae, A.; Checherita, I.A. Uric Acid and Oxidative Stress-Relationship with Cardiovascular, Metabolic, and Renal Impairment. *Int. J. Mol. Sci.* **2022**, *23*, 3188. [CrossRef]
40. Doria, A.; Galecki, A.T.; Spino, C.; Pop-Busui, R.; Cherney, D.Z.; Lingvay, I.; Parsa, A.; Rossing, P.; Sigal, R.J.; Afkarian, M.; et al. Serum Urate Lowering with Allopurinol and Kidney Function in Type 1 Diabetes. *N. Engl. J. Med.* **2020**, *382*, 2493–2503. [CrossRef]
41. Mauer, M.; Doria, A. Uric Acid and Diabetic Nephropathy Risk. *Contrib. Nephrol.* **2018**, *192*, 103–109. [CrossRef]
42. National Kidney Foundation. KDOQI Clinical Practice Guideline for Diabetes and CKD: 2012 Update. *Am. J. Kidney Dis.* **2012**, *60*, 850–886. [CrossRef]
43. La Grotta, R.; de Candia, P.; Olivieri, F.; Matacchione, G.; Giuliani, A.; Rippo, M.R.; Tagliabue, E.; Mancino, M.; Rispoli, F.; Ferroni, S.; et al. Anti-inflammatory effect of SGLT-2 inhibitors via uric acid and insulin. *Cell Mol. Life Sci.* **2022**, *79*, 273. [CrossRef]
44. Taderegew, M.M.; Gebremariam, T.; Tareke, A.A.; Woldeamanuel, G.G. Anemia and Its Associated Factors Among Type 2 Diabetes Mellitus Patients Attending Debre Berhan Referral Hospital, North-East Ethiopia: A Cross-Sectional Study. *J. Blood Med.* **2020**, *11*, 47–58. [CrossRef]
45. Solomon, D.; Bekele, K.; Atlaw, D.; Mamo, A.; Gezahegn, H.; Regasa, T.; Negash, G.; Nigussie, E.; Zenbaba, D.; Teferu, Z.; et al. Prevalence of anemia and associated factors among adult diabetic patients attending Bale zone hospitals, South-East Ethiopia. *PLoS ONE* **2022**, *17*, e0264007. [CrossRef]
46. Fujita, Y.; Doi, Y.; Hamano, T.; Hatazaki, M.; Umayahara, Y.; Isaka, Y.; Tsubakihara, Y. Low erythropoietin levels predict faster renal function decline in diabetic patients with anemia: A prospective cohort study. *Sci. Rep.* **2019**, *9*, 14871. [CrossRef]

47. AlDallal, S.M.; Jena, N. Prevalence of Anemia in Type 2 Diabetic Patients. *J. Hematol.* **2018**, *7*, 57–61. [CrossRef] [PubMed]
48. Kim, M.; Lee, S.H.; Park, K.S.; Kim, E.J.; Yeo, S.; Ha, I.H. Association between diabetes mellitus and anemia among Korean adults according to sex: A cross-sectional analysis of data from the Korea National Health and Nutrition Examination Survey (2010–2016). *BMC Endocr. Disord.* **2021**, *21*, 209. [CrossRef] [PubMed]
49. Nathwani, R.A.; Pais, S.; Reynolds, T.B.; Kaplowitz, N. Serum alanine aminotransferase in skeletal muscle diseases. *Hepatology* **2005**, *41*, 380–382. [CrossRef] [PubMed]
50. Malakouti, M.; Kataria, A.; Ali, S.K.; Schenker, S. Elevated Liver Enzymes in Asymptomatic Patients—What Should I Do? *J. Clin. Transl. Hepatol.* **2017**, *5*, 394–403. [CrossRef] [PubMed]
51. Mandal, A.; Bhattarai, B.; Kafle, P.; Khalid, M.; Jonnadula, S.K.; Lamicchane, J.; Kanth, R.; Gayam, V. Elevated Liver Enzymes in Patients with Type 2 Diabetes Mellitus and Non-alcoholic Fatty Liver Disease. *Cureus* **2018**, *10*, e3626. [CrossRef]
52. Muzurović, E.; van der Lely, A.J.; Gurnell, M. AST to ALT Ratio and Peripheral Arterial Disease in a Hypertensive Population—Is There a Link? *Angiology* **2021**, *72*, 905–907. [CrossRef]
53. Niu, H.; Zhou, Y. Nonlinear Relationship Between AST-to-ALT Ratio and the Incidence of Type 2 Diabetes Mellitus: A Follow-Up Study. *Int. J. Gen. Med.* **2021**, *14*, 8373–8382. [CrossRef]
54. Einarson, T.R.; Acs, A.; Ludwig, C.; Panton, U.H. Prevalence of cardiovascular disease in type 2 diabetes: A systematic literature review of scientific evidence from across the world in 2007-2017. *Cardiovasc. Diabetol.* **2018**, *17*, 83. [CrossRef]
55. Ma, C.X.; Ma, X.N.; Guan, C.H.; Li, Y.D.; Mauricio, D.; Fu, S.B. Cardiovascular disease in type 2 diabetes mellitus: Progress toward personalized management. *Cardiovasc. Diabetol.* **2022**, *21*, 74. [CrossRef]
56. Leon, B.M.; Maddox, T.M. Diabetes and cardiovascular disease: Epidemiology, biological mechanisms, treatment recommendations and future research. *World J. Diabetes* **2015**, *6*, 1246–1258. [CrossRef]
57. Matheus, A.S.; Tannus, L.R.; Cobas, R.A.; Palma, C.C.; Negrato, C.A.; Gomes, M.B. Impact of diabetes on cardiovascular disease: An update. *Int. J. Hypertens.* **2013**, *2013*, 653789. [CrossRef]
58. Cosentino, F.; Grant, P.J.; Aboyans, V.; Bailey, C.J.; Ceriello, A.; Delgado, V.; Federici, M.; Filippatos, G.; Grobbee, D.E.; Hansen, T.B.; et al. 2019 ESC Guidelines on diabetes, pre-diabetes, and cardiovascular diseases developed in collaboration with the EASD. *Eur. Heart. J.* **2020**, *41*, 255–323. [CrossRef]
59. Rawshani, A.; Rawshani, A.; Franzén, S.; Sattar, N.; Eliasson, B.; Svensson, A.M.; Zethelius, B.; Miftaraj, M.; McGuire, D.K.; Rosengren, A.; et al. Risk Factors, Mortality, and Cardiovascular Outcomes in Patients with Type 2 Diabetes. *N. Engl. J. Med.* **2018**, *379*, 633–644. [CrossRef]
60. Erqou, S.; Lee, C.T.; Suffoletto, M.; Echouffo-Tcheugui, J.B.; de Boer, R.A.; van Melle, J.P.; Adler, A.I. Association between glycated haemoglobin and the risk of congestive heart failure in diabetes mellitus: Systematic review and meta-analysis. *Eur. J. Heart Fail.* **2013**, *15*, 185–193. [CrossRef] [PubMed]
61. Penno, G.; Solini, A.; Zoppini, G.; Orsi, E.; Fondelli, C.; Zerbini, G.; Morano, S.; Cavalot, F.; Lamacchia, O.; Trevisan, R.; et al. Hemoglobin A1c variability as an independent correlate of cardiovascular disease in patients with type 2 diabetes: A cross-sectional analysis of the renal insufficiency and cardiovascular events (RIACE) Italian multicenter study. *Cardiovasc. Diabetol.* **2013**, *12*, 98. [CrossRef]
62. Huri, H.; Ling, D.; Ahmad, W.A. Association between glycemic control and antidiabetic drugs in type 2 diabetes mellitus patients with cardiovascular complications. *Drug Des. Devel. Ther.* **2015**, *9*, 4735–4749. [CrossRef]
63. Kenny, H.C.; Abel, E.D. Heart Failure in Type 2 Diabetes Mellitus. *Circ. Res.* **2019**, *124*, 121–141. [CrossRef]
64. Seferović, P.M.; Petrie, M.C.; Filippatos, G.S.; Anker, S.D.; Rosano, G.; Bauersachs, J.; Paulus, W.J.; Komajda, M.; Cosentino, F.; de Boer, R.A.; et al. Type 2 diabetes mellitus and heart failure: A position statement from the Heart Failure Association of the European Society of Cardiology. *Eur. J. Heart Fail.* **2018**, *20*, 853–872. [CrossRef]
65. Zinman, B.; Wanner, C.; Lachin, J.M.; Fitchett, D.; Bluhmki, E.; Hantel, S.; Mattheus, M.; Devins, T.; Johansen, O.E.; Woerle, H.J.; et al. Empagliflozin, Cardiovascular Outcomes, and Mortality in Type 2 Diabetes. *N. Engl. J. Med.* **2015**, *373*, 2117–2128. [CrossRef]
66. Neal, B.; Perkovic, V.; Matthews, D.R. Canagliflozin and Cardiovascular and Renal Events in Type 2 Diabetes. *N. Engl. J. Med.* **2017**, *377*, 2099. [CrossRef]
67. Wiviott, S.D.; Raz, I.; Bonaca, M.P.; Mosenzon, O.; Kato, E.T.; Cahn, A.; Silverman, M.G.; Zelniker, T.A.; Kuder, J.F.; Murphy, S.A.; et al. Dapagliflozin and Cardiovascular Outcomes in Type 2 Diabetes. *N. Engl. J. Med.* **2019**, *380*, 347–357. [CrossRef] [PubMed]
68. Silva-Cardoso, J.; Andrade, A.; Brito, D.; Ferreira, J.; Fonseca, C.; Peres, M.; Franco, F.; Moura, B. SGLT-2 inhibitors: A step forward in the treatment of heart failure with reduced ejection fraction. *Rev. Port. Cardiol. (Engl. Ed.)* **2021**, *40*, 687–693. [CrossRef] [PubMed]
69. Richardson, T.L., Jr.; Hackstadt, A.J.; Hung, A.M.; Greevy, R.A.; Grijalva, C.G.; Griffin, M.R.; Elasy, T.A.; Roumie, C.L. Hospitalization for Heart Failure Among Patients With Diabetes Mellitus and Reduced Kidney Function Treated With Metformin Versus Sulfonylureas: A Retrospective Cohort Study. *J. Am. Heart Assoc.* **2021**, *10*, e019211. [CrossRef] [PubMed]
70. Leiter, L.A. Latest Evidence on Sulfonylureas: What's New? *Diabetes Ther.* **2020**, *11* (Suppl. 1), 15–22. [CrossRef] [PubMed]
71. Wijnen, M.; Duschek, E.J.J.; Boom, H.; van Vliet, M. The effects of antidiabetic agents on heart failure. *Neth. Heart J.* **2022**, *30*, 65–75. [CrossRef]

72. Gembillo, G.; Ingrasciotta, Y.; Crisafulli, S.; Luxi, N.; Siligato, R.; Santoro, D.; Trifirò, G. Kidney Disease in Diabetic Patients: From Pathophysiology to Pharmacological Aspects with a Focus on Therapeutic Inertia. *Int. J. Mol. Sci.* **2021**, *22*, 4824. [CrossRef]
73. Xu, Y.; Surapaneni, A.; Alkas, J.; Evans, M.; Shin, J.I.; Selvin, E.; Chang, A.; Grams, M.E.; Carrero, J.J. Glycemic Control and the Risk of Acute Kidney Injury in Patients With Type 2 Diabetes and Chronic Kidney Disease: Parallel Population-Based Cohort Studies in U.S. and Swedish Routine Care. *Diabetes Care* **2020**, *43*, 2975–2982. [CrossRef]
74. Vart, P.; Correa-Rotter, R.; Hou, F.F.; Jongs, N.; Chertow, G.M.; Langkilde, A.M.; McMurray, J.J.V.; Rossing p Sjöström, C.D.; Stefansson, B.V.; Toto, R.D.; et al. Efficacy and Safety of Dapagliflozin in Patients With CKD Across Major Geographic Regions. *Kidney Int. Rep.* **2022**, *7*, 699–707. [CrossRef]
75. Song, A.; Zhang, C.; Meng, X. Mechanism and application of metformin in kidney diseases: An update. *Biomed. Pharmacother.* **2021**, *138*, 111454. [CrossRef]
76. De Broe, M.E.; Kajbaf, F.; Lalau, J.D. Renoprotective Effects of Metformin. *Nephron* **2018**, *138*, 261–274. [CrossRef]
77. Chaudhury, A.; Duvoor, C.; Reddy Dendi, V.S.; Kraleti, S.; Chada, A.; Ravilla, R.; Marco, A.; Shekhawat, N.S.; Montales, M.T.; Kuriakose, K.; et al. Clinical Review of Antidiabetic Drugs: Implications for Type 2 Diabetes Mellitus Management. *Front. Endocrinol.* **2017**, *8*, 6. [CrossRef]
78. Cianciolo, G.; De Pascalis, A.; Capelli, I.; Gasperoni, L.; Di Lullo, L.; Bellasi, A.; La Manna, G. Mineral and Electrolyte Disorders With SGLT2i Therapy. *JBMR Plus* **2019**, *3*, e10242. [CrossRef]
79. Baker, C.; Retzik-Stahr, C.; Singh, V.; Plomondon, R.; Anderson, V.; Rasouli, N. Should metformin remain the first-line therapy for treatment of type 2 diabetes? *Ther. Adv. Endocrinol. Metab.* **2021**, *12*, 2042018820980225. [CrossRef]
80. Ober, S.K.; Watts, S.; Lawrence, R.H. Insulin use in elderly diabetic patients. *Clin. Interv. Aging* **2006**, *1*, 107–113. [CrossRef]
81. Pedrosa, M.R.; Franco, D.R.; Gieremek, H.W.; Vidal, C.M.; Bronzeri, F.; de Cassia Rocha, A.; de Carvalho Cara, L.G.; Fogo, S.L.; Eliaschewitz, F.G. GLP-1 Agonist to Treat Obesity and Prevent Cardiovascular Disease: What Have We Achieved so Far? *Curr. Atheroscler. Rep.* **2022**, *24*, 867–884. [CrossRef]
82. Dennis, J.M.; Henley, W.E.; Weedon, M.N.; Lonergan, M.; Rodgers, L.R.; Jones, A.G.; Hamilton, W.T.; Sattar, N.; Janmohamed, S.; Holman, R.R.; et al. Sex and BMI Alter the Benefits and Risks of Sulfonylureas and Thiazolidinediones in Type 2 Diabetes: A Framework for Evaluating Stratification Using Routine Clinical and Individual Trial Data. *Diabetes Care* **2018**, *41*, 1844–1853. [CrossRef]
83. Custódio, J.S., Jr.; Roriz-Filho, J.; Cavalcanti, C.A.J.; Martins, A.; Salles, J.E.N. Use of SGLT2 Inhibitors in Older Adults: Scientific Evidence and Practical Aspects. *Drugs Aging* **2020**, *37*, 399–409. [CrossRef]
84. Lee, W.C.; Balu, S.; Cobden, D.; Joshi, A.V.; Pashos, C.L. Medication adherence and the associated health-economic impact among patients with type 2 diabetes mellitus converting to insulin pen therapy: An analysis of third-party managed care claims data. *Clin. Ther.* **2006**, *28*, 1712–1725. [CrossRef] [PubMed]
85. Pollack, M.F.; Purayidathil, F.W.; Bolge, S.C.; Williams, S.A. Patient-reported tolerability issues with oral antidiabetic agents: Associations with adherence; treatment satisfaction and health-related quality of life. *Diabetes Res. Clin. Pract.* **2010**, *87*, 204–210. [CrossRef]
86. Jin, J.; Sklar, G.E.; Min Sen Oh, V.; Chuen Li, S. Factors affecting therapeutic compliance: A review from the patient's perspective. *Ther. Clin. Risk Manag.* **2008**, *4*, 269–286. [CrossRef]
87. Wong, M.C.; Kong, A.P.; So, W.Y.; Jiang, J.Y.; Chan, J.C.; Griffiths, S.M. Adherence to oral hypoglycemic agents in 26,782 Chinese patients: A cohort study. *J. Clin. Pharmacol.* **2011**, *51*, 1474–1482. [CrossRef] [PubMed]
88. Akash, G.; Shwetha, B.; Basavaraj, C.K.; Chetan, A.C. Drug utilization pattern in type II diabetes mellitus patients attending non-communicable disease clinic in a tertiary care hospital. *Int. J. Basic Clin. Pharmacol.* **2019**, *8*, 539–544. [CrossRef]
89. Orlando, V.; Guerriero, F.; Putignano, D.; Monetti, V.M.; Tari, D.U.; Farina, G.; Illario, M.; Iaccarino, G.; Menditto, E. Prescription Patterns of Antidiabetic Treatment in the Elderly. Results from Southern Italy. *Curr. Diabetes Rev.* **2015**, *12*, 100–106. [CrossRef] [PubMed]
90. Hutchins, V.; Zhang, B.; Fleurence, R.L.; Krishnarajah, G.; Graham, J. A systematic review of adherence, treatment satisfaction and costs, in fixed-dose combination regimens in type 2 diabetes. *Curr. Med. Res. Opin.* **2011**, *27*, 1157–1168. [CrossRef] [PubMed]
91. Bagonza, J.; Rutebemberwa, E.; Bazeyo, W. Adherence to anti diabetic medication among patients with diabetes in eastern Uganda; a cross sectional study. *BMC Health Serv. Res.* **2015**, *15*, 168. [CrossRef]
92. Lunati, M.E.; Cimino, V.; Gandolfi, A.; Trevisan, M.; Montefusco, L.; Pastore, I.; Pace, C.; Betella, N.; Favacchio, G.; Bulgheroni, M.; et al. SGLT2-inhibitors are effective and safe in the elderly: The SOLD study. *Pharmacol. Res.* **2022**, *183*, 106396. [CrossRef]
93. Fang, H.S.A.; Gao, Q.; Tan, W.Y.; Lee, M.L.; Hsu, W.; Tan, N.C. The effect of oral diabetes medications on glycated haemoglobin (HbA1c) in Asians in primary care: A retrospective cohort real-world data study. *BMC Med.* **2022**, *20*, 22. [CrossRef]
94. Palanisamy, S.; Yien, E.L.H.; Shi, L.W.; Si, L.Y.; Qi, S.H.; Ling, L.S.C.; Lun, T.W.; Chen, Y.N. Systematic Review of Efficacy and Safety of Newer Antidiabetic Drugs Approved from 2013 to 2017 in Controlling HbA1c in Diabetes Patients. *Pharmacy* **2018**, *6*, 57. [CrossRef]
95. Mearns, E.S.; Sobieraj, D.M.; White, C.M.; Saulsberry, W.J.; Kohn, C.G.; Doleh, Y.; Zaccaro, E.; Coleman, C.I. Comparative efficacy and safety of antidiabetic drug regimens added to metformin monotherapy in patients with type 2 diabetes: A network meta-analysis. *PLoS ONE* **2015**, *10*, e0125879. [CrossRef]

96. Peng, Y.; Chen, S.H.; Liu, X.N.; Sun, Q.Y. Efficacy of different antidiabetic drugs based on metformin in the treatment of type 2 diabetes mellitus: A network meta-analysis involving eight eligible randomized-controlled trials. *J. Cell Physiol.* **2019**, *234*, 2795–2806. [CrossRef]
97. Chamberlain, J.J.; Rhinehart, A.S.; Shaefer, C.F., Jr.; Neuman, A. Diagnosis and Management of Diabetes: Synopsis of the 2016 American Diabetes Association Standards of Medical Care in Diabetes. *Ann. Intern. Med.* **2016**, *164*, 542–552. [CrossRef]
98. Dahlén, A.D.; Dashi, G.; Maslov, I.; Attwood, M.M.; Jonsson, J.; Trukhan, V.; Schiöth, H.B. Trends in Antidiabetic Drug Discovery: FDA Approved Drugs, New Drugs in Clinical Trials and Global Sales. *Front. Pharmacol.* **2022**, *12*, 807548. [CrossRef]
99. van den Boom, L.; Kaiser, M.; Kostev, K. Prevalence of insulin as a first-line therapy and associated factors in people with type 2 diabetes in German primary care practices. *Diabetes Med.* **2020**, *37*, 1333–1339. [CrossRef]
100. Lebovitz, H.E. Insulin: Potential negative consequences of early routine use in patients with type 2 diabetes. *Diabetes Care* **2011**, *34* (Suppl. 2), S225–S230. [CrossRef]
101. Piera-Mardemootoo, C.; Lambert, P.; Faillie, J.L. Efficacy of metformin on glycemic control and weight in drug-naive type 2 diabetes mellitus patients: A systematic review and meta-analysis of placebo-controlled randomized trials. *Therapie* **2021**, *76*, 647–656. [CrossRef]
102. Hostalek, U.; Gwilt, M.; Hildemann, S. Therapeutic Use of Metformin in Prediabetes and Diabetes Prevention. *Drugs* **2015**, *75*, 1071–1094. [CrossRef]
103. Sola, D.; Rossi, L.; Schianca, G.P.; Maffioli, P.; Bigliocca, M.; Mella, R.; Corlianò, F.; Fra, G.P.; Bartoli, E.; Derosa, G. Sulfonylureas and their use in clinical practice. *Arch. Med. Sci.* **2015**, *11*, 840–848. [CrossRef]
104. Rao, A.D.; Kuhadiya, N.; Reynolds, K.; Fonseca, V.A. Is the combination of sulfonylureas and metformin associated with an increased risk of cardiovascular disease or all-cause mortality?: A meta-analysis of observational studies. *Diabetes Care* **2008**, *31*, 1672–1678. [CrossRef]
105. Schramm, T.K.; Gislason, G.H.; Vaag, A.; Rasmussen, J.N.; Folke, F.; Hansen, M.L.; Fosbøl, E.L.; Køber, L.; Norgaard, M.L.; Madsen, M.; et al. Mortality and cardiovascular risk associated with different insulin secretagogues compared with metformin in type 2 diabetes, with or without a previous myocardial infarction: A nationwide study. *Eur. Heart J.* **2011**, *32*, 1900–1908. [CrossRef]
106. Pop, L.M.; Lingvay, I. The Infamous, Famous Sulfonylureas and Cardiovascular Safety: Much Ado About Nothing? *Curr. Diab. Rep.* **2017**, *17*, 124. [CrossRef]
107. Chai, S.; Zhang, R.; Zhang, Y.; Carr, R.D.; Zheng, Y.; Rajpathak, S.; Yu, M. Influence of dipeptidyl peptidase-4 inhibitors on glycemic variability in patients with type 2 diabetes: A meta-analysis of randomized controlled trials. *Front. Endocrinol.* **2022**, *13*, 935039. [CrossRef] [PubMed]
108. Kang, S.M.; Park, J.H. Pleiotropic Benefits of DPP-4 Inhibitors Beyond Glycemic Control. *Clin. Med. Insights Endocrinol. Diabetes* **2021**, *14*, 11795514211051698. [CrossRef]
109. Nauck, M.A.; Quast, D.R. Cardiovascular Safety and Benefits of Semaglutide in Patients With Type 2 Diabetes: Findings From SUSTAIN 6 and PIONEER 6. *Front. Endocrinol.* **2021**, *12*, 645566. [CrossRef]
110. Rowlands, J.; Heng, J.; Newsholme, P.; Carlessi, R. Pleiotropic Effects of GLP-1 and Analogs on Cell Signaling, Metabolism, and Function. *Front. Endocrinol.* **2018**, *9*, 672. [CrossRef] [PubMed]
111. Pirklbauer, M.; Schupart, R.; Fuchs, L.; Staudinger, P.; Corazza, U.; Sallaberger, S.; Leierer, J.; Mayer, G.; Schramek, H. Unraveling reno-protective effects of SGLT2 inhibition in human proximal tubular cells. *Am. J. Physiol. Renal. Physiol.* **2019**, *316*, F449–F462. [CrossRef] [PubMed]
112. Ni, L.; Yuan, C.; Chen, G.; Zhang, C.; Wu, X. SGLT2i: Beyond the glucose-lowering effect. *Cardiovasc. Diabetol.* **2020**, *19*, 98. [CrossRef]
113. Unnikrishnan, R.; Anjana, R.M.; Deepa, M.; Pradeepa, R.; Joshi, S.R.; Bhansali, A.; Dhandania, V.K.; Joshi, P.P.; Madhu, S.V.; Rao, P.V.; et al. Glycemic control among individuals with self-reported diabetes in India–the ICMR-INDIAB Study. *Diabetes Technol. Ther.* **2014**, *16*, 596–603. [CrossRef]
114. Gebrie, D.; Manyazewal, T.; AEjigu, D.; Makonnen, E. Metformin-Insulin versus Metformin-Sulfonylurea Combination Therapies in Type 2 Diabetes: A Comparative Study of Glycemic Control and Risk of Cardiovascular Diseases in Addis Ababa, Ethiopia. *Diabetes Metab. Syndr. Obes.* **2021**, *14*, 3345–3359. [CrossRef]
115. Ling, S.; Zaccardi, F.; Lawson, C.; Seidu, S.I.; Davies, M.J.; Khunti, K. Glucose Control, Sulfonylureas, and Insulin Treatment in Elderly People With Type 2 Diabetes and Risk of Severe Hypoglycemia and Death: An Observational Study. *Diabetes Care* **2021**, *44*, 915–924. [CrossRef]
116. Vedantam, D.; Poman, D.S.; Motwani, L.; Asif, N.; Patel, A.; Anne, K.K. Stress-Induced Hyperglycemia: Consequences and Management. *Cureus* **2022**, *14*, e26714. [CrossRef]
117. Xiu, F.; Stanojcic, M.; Diao, L.; Jeschke, M.G. Stress Hyperglycemia, Insulin Treatment, and Innate Immune Cells. *Int. J. Endocrinol.* **2014**, *2014*, 486403. [CrossRef]

MDPI AG
Grosspeteranlage 5
4052 Basel
Switzerland
Tel.: +41 61 683 77 34

Biomedicines Editorial Office
E-mail: biomedicines@mdpi.com
www.mdpi.com/journal/biomedicines

www.ingramcontent.com/pod-product-compliance
Lightning Source LLC
Chambersburg PA
CBHW062102220926
51850CB00010B/2862
9783725867660